MOTOR DEVELOPMENT

Anna S. Espenschade
Helen M. Eckert

University of California
Berkeley, California

CHARLES E. MERRILL PUBLISHING CO.
Columbus, Ohio

Library of Congress Catalog Number: 67-20932

6 7 8 9 10 11 12 13 —
75 74 73

ISBN 0-675-09738-X

Printed in the United States of America

PREFACE

There is an impressive body of knowledge relating to motor development and motor performance, especially in the very early years of life. It comes from many disciplines, each tending to approach it from a different viewpoint and to incorporate findings into a discipline-related complex. Thus the student of motor development per se must search far and wide for sources.

No one book can hope to include all of the knowledge in this area. In this one the authors have attempted to trace the outline of growth and decline, to describe some of the methods and the problems of investigators and to point out the paucity of information in certain areas.

Physical educators, physical therapists and others with a biological background will be especially interested in the growth processes themselves and in the interrelationships of structure and function. Psychologists and educators, as students of behavior, will find physical and motor development important variables in human actions and interactions.

This book is designed to serve as a text for undergraduate students and as a source book for more advanced students who may wish to follow up references in various areas. The authors acknowledge their indebtedness to the many students who have intentionally or otherwise served as judges for the selection of the content of this volume.

Anna S. Espenschade

Helen M. Eckert

iii

CONTENTS

        CHILDHOOD   137

        Changes in Size and Body Proportions, 138
        Indices of Growth and Maturation, 139
        Body Build, 144
        Growth and Maturation Indices and Motor
            Performance, 148
        Development of Strength, 150
        Changes in Motor Performance, 157
            a. running
            b. jumping
            c. throwing
            d. flexibility
            e. balance
            f. coordination
            g. general
        Interest and Motor Activity, 169

IX   ADOLESCENT DEVELOPMENT   173

        Factors Affecting Onset of Puberty, 179
        Factors Affecting Puberal Growth Spurt, 181
        Seasonal Variation in Growth, 186
        Changes in Body Proportions, 188
        Physiological Changes, 193
        Changes in Body Tissues, 205
        Strength Increments, 206
        Changes in Motor Performance, 210
        Motor Coordination and Balance, 215
        Secular Trends and Geographic Variation in
            Motor Performance, 218

CHAPTER I

HEREDITY

Each individual receives from his parents the greatest gift of all—that of life. Through the parents come also a multiplicity of hereditary factors which determine to a great extent physical appearance and maximum potential. Environment from the moment of conception modifies and interacts with heredity to shape the individual and to control the extent to which the maximal potential will be realized. It is difficult, if not impossible, to assess the relative contributions of heredity and environment.

The great variability of physical appearances in the general population is obvious from a casual observation of persons encountered during a short walk down any busy street. Family resemblances are consistently present, however, and are a continuing source of interest. A boy may be the "image of his father," or perhaps he looks more like his mother or older brothers. If the offspring are identical twins, observers have the impression of seeing double. The duplication of what appears to be one individual has proven to be a fruitful model for research into the relative effects of heredity and environment. Such studies indicate that physical characteristics are determined to a great extent by heredity and are little affected by environment.

It is obvious that a child deprived of adequate food and shelter may be harmed physically. It is becoming increasingly evident that in our society no one can attain his maximal potential in any respect if he does not grow up under favorable conditions. Children of parents of high intelligence tend to show higher intelligence than children of parents of low intelligence. At the same time, children of professional groups and those of higher socio-economic status have the highest IQ's while children of unskilled laborers have the lowest. Relationships between the IQ's of the child and the socio-economic status of the parents tend to increase with the age of the child. Maximal potential in intelligence is determined by heredity but the extent to which it is achieved is limited by environment.

Human abilities and characteristics most affected by environment prove to be the ones in which increasing differences are observed as individuals grow older. Beliefs, values, and attitudes in which training and proximity are major factors have little or no hereditary basis. Temperamental characteristics in which glandular activity may be involved are somewhat dependent upon heredity. Scheinfeld (1939) indicates that intelligence, sensory discrimination, speed of reaction, and motor coordinations are among those facets of human behavior determined to a great extent by heredity.

THEORIES OF HEREDITY

The inheritance of parental traits by offspring has fascinated man from earliest times and there are many indications that attempts were made to influence heredity by selective breeding. The numerous strains of dogs extant today indicate the degree to which our ancestors were successful in breeding the types of animals best suited to their needs. Attention to the details of breeding in ancient times is indicated by a Babylonian stone tablet, evacuated in Chaldea and dated at approximately 4000 B.C., which shows the inheritance of head and mane characteristics in five generations of horses. Flora as well as fauna have been selectively bred to develop varieties more suitable to human needs. Archeologists have associated the improved yield of grains and maize with the rise of ancient civilizations. Early Chinese accounts indicate that superior varieties of rice were developed almost 6,000 years ago, while ancient Egyptian paintings depict men cross-pollinating the date palm (Winchester, 1961).

Until relatively recently, human offspring were considered a mixture of the blood of their parents and hereditary traits were believed to be passed on in this blended blood from the parents. Hence the common referrals in literature to the blood of some renowned ancestor "flowing" in the veins of the hero or heroine. We still tend to use the term "blue blood" to refer to individuals who have a royal or noble ancestry although it is common knowledge that all blood is the same color and that blood is a product of each individual's body with not even a mother and her child having a single drop of blood in common.

Another inheritance theory that has been expressed in the past is the so-called "jig-saw" method of race inheritance whereby, for example, a child may be ¼ Scotch, ⅛ Irish, ⅛ French, ¼ Italian, and other, and, of course, inherit frugality from his Scotch ancestors, emotionality from the French and Italian, and so forth. Scheinfeld (1939) gives a very succinct and realistic appraisal of the futility of assigning characteristics to races while genetics, the modern study of heredity, makes it very clear that each offspring is an individual identity and not so many parts of this and that.

MENDELIAN LAWS

A Moravian monk, Gregor Mendel, working with garden peas, discovered three relationships which have become the cornerstones of research in the field of genetics. The conclusions drawn by Mendel have since been referred to as the "Mendelian laws" of genetics and in modern terminology may be stated as follows:

1. Inherited characteristics are carried by genes which are passed along unchanged from one generation to another.
2. Genes are found in pairs in each individual. The two genes in a pair may be different in their effects and where this occurs,

one gene tends to dominate the other, in which case it is referred to as the "dominant" while the other is known as the
"recessive."

3. When reproductive cells are formed in any individual by the
process of reduction division, the genes in each pair separate
with only one of each pair going to each reproductive cell.

REPRODUCTIVE CELL DIVISION

A glance at the actual mechanism of meiosis, or reproductive cell
division, indicates the complexities which stand in the way of any
accurate predictions of the offspring of human parents. It has been
clearly established that the normal human being has 46 chromosomes in the nucleus of the cell. The 46 chromosomes are made up
of varying numbers of genes which are fixed in their effect and, in
44 of these chromosomes, there are pairs, or alleles, of each of the
genes that work together as single units in the effect that is produced, e.g., the action of paired dominant and recessive genes. In
the female the remaining two chromosomes are also paired while, in
the male, the Y chromosome is much shorter than the X chromosome so that a number of the X genes remain unpaired.

Normal body growth requires that cell division occur and also
requires that the cells be duplicated in their entirety if the integrity
of the structure is to be maintained. During the normal process of
cell division, or mitosis, the number of chromosomes in the cell is
the same before and after division. Reproduction, however, requires
that the chromosomal number be reduced in half to allow for equal
chromosomal contributions by each parent to the offspring.

Figure 1 illustrates, by the use of 6 chromosomes, how the diploid
number of chromosomes (46) is reduced to the haploid number (23)
with the maturation of the germ cells during the process of oögenesis
(egg formation) and spermatogenesis (sperm formation). During the
first step, or prophase, of meiosis there is a pairing of chromosomes
with their homologous mates which is not present in the prophase
of mitosis. By the time pairing is completed, the chromonemata,
but not the centromere, of each chromosome has been duplicated to
form two chromatids attached to the single centromere. It is at this
time that the paired chromosomes may become entangled and a
"cross-over" occur in the genes of the chromosomes.

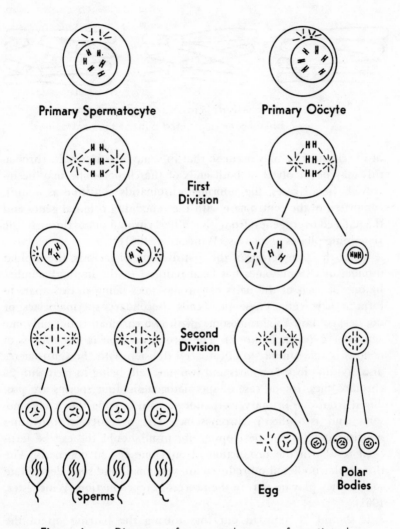

Figure 1.   Diagram of egg and sperm formation by
                  meiosis.

The mechanism of crossing over in two paired chromosomes is
illustrated in Figure 2, where overlapping of one of the chromatids
of each pair results in an interchange of the genes between the
overlapped segments. Any amount of overlapping and interchange

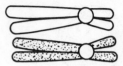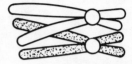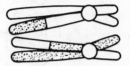

Figure 2.   Mechanism of crossing over. The chromonemata
                  have been duplicated but not the centromere.

of the chromatids may occur so that in some instances both chromatids may be involved or both ends of the chromosome may be involved. In all cases, the reformed chromatids continue as a unit,
comprised of the centromere with the remaining original genes and
the crossed-over genes from the other chromosome, through the
remaining phases of meiosis (Winchester, 1961).

Upon the completion of the first division of meiosis, the diploid
number of chromosomes has been reduced to the haploid number
by one of each of the pairs of chromosomes being drawn apart to
form a new cell. These new cells (secondary spermatocytes or
oöcytes) contain 23 chromosomes with two chromatids but only one
centromere (as in Figure 2). The second division in the process of
meiosis is very similar to mitotic cell division with the centromeres
also dividing into two parts and two new cells being formed with 23
chromosomes. In the case of spermatogenesis, four sperms are produced from one primary spermatocyte, two bearing the X chromosome and two the Y chromosome. The necessity of providing
nourishment for the developing organism should the egg be fertilized results in the production of only one egg in oögenesis. The
three polar bodies also produced are very small and soon degenerate
so that they play no part in the process of reproduction (Winchester,
1961).

It should be pointed out that during the pairing up of the
chromosomes in the prophase of meiosis such pairings are done in
a haphazard manner with respect to the relative position of the
pairs in relation to each other. That is, all the chromosomes inherited from the father do not line up on the right side while those
from the mother do so on the left, or vice versa. Thus the offspring
may inherit a chromosome from the first pair from his mother, the

next from his father, and so on, in any combination of dual arrangement of the 23 pairs. Moreover, it should be noted that the arrangement of the 23 pairs will probably be different in every germ cell during the course of its meiotic division. To this staggering number of possible combinations one must add the consideration that crossing over may have occurred in genes while each chromosome of a pair was composed of two chromatids, and, further, that this crossing over may occur in any amount in any of the paired chromosomes. Within just a single pair of genes of a pair of chromosomes there are, as will be seen below in the case of brachyphalangy, four possible combinations. It is now estimated that there are approximately 50,000 genes in the 46 chromosomes, with the odds being about 1 in 200,000 trillion that the same parents will ever present the same packet of chromosomes to another child (Hicks, 1963). It is small wonder, then, that our prediction of the characteristics of human offspring is very unreliable, and we must content ourselves with the very general conclusion that heredity does tend to create likenesses in families.

GENETIC COMPOSITION

How, we may ask, do the genes regulate and order the growth and division of one single cell to eventually become the 26 trillion multidifferentiated, interrelated, and integrated cells that form the small human organism that we commonly call a baby? Unfortunately, very little is known about this process. We do know, however, that the hereditary blueprint governing the functions of all cells is embodied in the molecules of deoxyribonucleic. acid (DNA) which are built up in an ordered linear sequence of nucleotids containing the same four bases in two linked pairs; namely, the base adenine paired with thymine and guanine paired with cytosine. The classic gene, therefore, containing a number of these nucleotides which may occur in different proportions within the units of the DNA chain, has great numbers of combinational possibilities in its subgenic structure whereby it may transmit information. It is hypothesized that the actual transmission of information is accomplished through the intermediates of ribonucleic acids (RNA) or ribonucleoproteins, which are believed to act as messengers carrying the "code" for protein synthesis from the DNA chain to the areas in which the protein is to be synthesized. The possibility that RNA may serve as a template is supported by the similarity of its biochemical structure to that of DNA, with the thymine in the latter being replaced by the base uracil in the former and by RNA's intermediate position between DNA and protein formation in the gene-protein action system (Waddington, 1962). The close coupling of the gene-protein action system is supported by biochemical analyses of certain gene mutations, which have indicated an alteration of only one amino acid in the linear sequence of a protein which may contain as many as a hundred or more such links within the whole molecule (Waddington, 1962).

Recently, Sager (1965) has reported the existence of nonchromosomal genes carrying primary genetic information and cites work of David J. L. Luck and Edward Reich of the Rockefeller Institute which demonstrated the localization of extranuclear DNA in mitochondria, a feature common to all plant and animal cells. These findings indicate additional sources other than the chromosomes for transmitting the genetic information necessary for morphogenic development, and may play an important part in time differences and rate differences as well as in organelle differences in development. Considering the vast number of changes necessary in the developmental sequence whereby a single fertilized ovum eventually becomes a fully matured human being, embryologists have questioned the possibility of such a vast storage of knowledge within the relatively small confines of 46 chromosomes. Moreover, different structural complexes appear at different times and with different rates of development; nor do they appear in full bloom but often require many adjustments before achieving their ultimate form.

Waddington (1962) points out that the cytoplasm of the ovum is not a homogeneous mass but contains many different types of protein which are in constant interaction as evidenced by the streaming of cytoplasmic material seen under a microscope. He contends that a certain amount of differentiation may occur in the ovum on the basis of the initial spatial distribution of these interactions with respect to the polarity of the cell. In the morphogenesis of masses containing large numbers of cells, Waddington (1962) indicates that the interactions of the chemicals of the cell membranes and the formation of attachment bodies, or desmosomes, may give rise to the mechanisms whereby the unification of the structure is achieved. Both of these types of interaction would require a feedback type of system rather than a one-way circuitry for effective operation. Similarly, if the gene-protein system incorporates some mechanism of feedback, an explanation is forthcoming for the ordered development of complex systems with different rates of development and in various time sequences. Waddington (1962) has postulated the existence of such a system which he has termed the "gene-action system" within which are incorporated short series of reactions leading from the gene to the first protein it determines and labelled "gene-protein systems." Feedback from the gene-protein system, which in turn is in interaction with the cytoplasm, influences the gene-action system of which it is a part. Since the genes themselves are constantly interacting with one another, the feedback from the gene-protein system may result in inter-genetic adjustments or serve as confirmation that "all is progressing as scheduled." Such an arrangement obviously incorporates a greater range of possibilities in the transmission of genetic information than a one-way copying system and also allows for minor deviations and variabilities from a set pattern for adjustment to external influences.

Glass (Shock, 1960) would seem to support the concept of genetic interaction, for he points to the abundant evidence from studies of suppressor genes indicating that the action of a particular gene may be turned on or off, without the gene itself being modified, by the action of a gene at another locus. He believes that this may be accomplished by controlling the flow of a limited amount of substrate through competing channels or by the provision of an alternate route, or bypass, for the formation of the chemical product of the particular gene-controlled reaction. Glass draws the conclusion that there is much evidence to support the theory that differentiation proceeds by controls over gene activity without altering the ultimate nature of the gene itself. This would seem to be a very sound point of view, since the fertilized ovum, along with a limited amount of protein, contains only chromosomes comprised of the genes and the genes must remain unchanged throughout the division and differentiation process to become the continuing part of the germ cells which will eventually mature into gametes in preparation for the production of the next generation of off-spring.

DOMINANT AND RECESSIVE GENES

Despite the extreme complication of the genetic transmission process, we are, because of the dominant and recessive relationship between some pairs of genes, able to make reasonably accurate predictions of certain characteristics. In human beings, dominant and recessive genes control such physical features as eye shape and color, length of eye lashes, ear lobe attachment and size of ear, nose shape, hair texture and color, thickness of lip, and stature.

In some instances, the pairing of two recessive genes will produce a lethal combination resulting in deatn in early infancy. Such "killer" genes have been identified as producing glioma retina (eye tumor), amaurotic family idiocy, malignant freckles, and progressive spinal muscular atrophy in infants (Scheinfeld, 1939). Some dominant genes may be "intermediate lethals" in humans as they may pair with a recessive gene to produce nothing more than an abnormal effect, whereas the pairing of two such dominant genes will result in death. Such a gene exists for brachyphalangy, a condition in which the middle joint of the fingers is greatly shortened. A marriage between two individuals having this condition resulted in one of the four children, which was unable to survive, being born without any fingers or toes and with other skeletal defects. Of the surviving three children, one had normal fingers while the other two possessed short fingers. The exact 1:2:1 ratio was what could be expected if one considered the short fingers as being an intermediate expression of a dominant lethal gene (Winchester, 1961). A graphic illustration of this type of situation is presented in Figure 3.

With brachyphalangy being produced by a dominant gene and the ratio of 2:1 tending to exist in surviving children of parents who both have brachyphalangy, one might well question why the abnormality is not more common. It is entirely possible that an individual with short fingers might have been so handicapped during the periods in our cultural development when physical skill was a prerequisite to survival that few of them lived to reproduce. On the other hand, it is possible that brachyphalangy may be a relatively

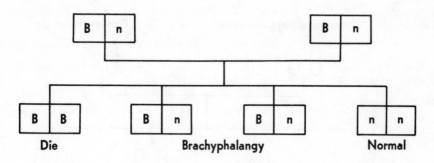

Figure 3.   Distribution of children from a marriage of two
individuals with brachyphalangy.

recent genetic mutation, in which case the possibility of marriage
between two people having the condition is not very great and the
ratio of brachyphalangy in the children of a marriage involving
only one person with brachyphalangy would tend to be 2:2. In any
event, it is quite likely that this and other genetic abnormalities will
tend to increase in the future due to the advances in medical science
which enable increasing numbers to survive.

SEX-LINKED GENES

The foregoing discussion of dominant and recessive genes applies
to all the paired genes in 44 of the 46 chromosomes in the human
body. The remaining two chromosomes are the sex determinants of
an individual and are called the X and Y chromosomes. The X
chromosome has been found to be much longer than the Y chromosome which means that a number of the genes in the X chromosome are unpaired in the male of the species (XY chromosome
arrangement). As the X chromosome in the male comes from the
mother, the son inherits all the effects of these unmatched genes
regardless of whether they would be dominant or recessive in a pairing with the genes of another X chromosome.

Figure 4 illustrates the transmission of color blindness from
mother to son while the daughters, although also having a color
blind gene, do not have the symptoms because, since the gene is
recessive, its effect is masked by the dominant color vision gene.

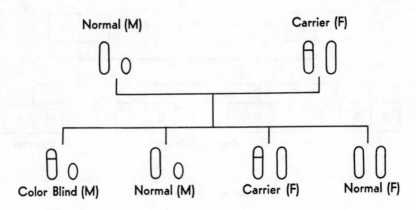

Normal (M)   Carrier (F)

Color Blind (M)   Normal (M)   Carrier (F)   Normal (F)

Figure 4.   Diagram of transmission of color blindness in humans.

Only in the rare instance of a marriage between a color blind man and a woman with a recessive color gene, or even rarer, with a color blind woman, would there be color blind female children. The same explanation applies to the other major sex-linked abnormality, hemophelia. In this latter instance, however, where records indicate the presence of hemophelia in women, it seems to manifest itself in a variation in the degree of blood clotting rather than in the complete absence of clotting. It would seem that the female function of childbearing requires that no one gene have an excessive dominance in this area if the species is to survive (Winchester, 1961). Perhaps the effect of the "baldness" gene which is called a sex-limited gene, more closely approximates the action of the gene producing hemophelia. The "baldness" gene is a dominant in men with only one being required to produce baldness while in women the gene acts as a recessive with two being necessary to produce even partial baldness (Scheinfeld, 1939)

SEX RATIO AND MORTALITY

The imbalance of genes in the X and Y chromosomes seems to have effects beyond the determination of the sex of the individual with its numerous ramifications of biological sex development. In looking at the sex of live births in the United States, an excess of males over females is found that could not be due to chance since our knowledge of meiosis indicates the production of an equal number of sperms with X and Y chromosomes by the male parent. One theory in explanation of this phenomenon is that, since the Y chromosome is smaller than the X chromosome, the sperms carrying the Y are lighter in weight and smaller in size giving them a slight advantage in the race for the egg or, perhaps, an advantage in penetrating the egg should both Y and X bearing sperms arrive at the egg at the same time (Winchester, 1961).

Although the sex ratio favors the male, 106 to 100 at birth, the sexes are nearly equal in number at 20 years of age. Later in life, women outnumber men by about 100 to 85 at the age of 50 and at 85 years of age are twice as numerous as men. Some people contend that the pressures of modern life are more rigorous for men than women hence the higher mortality rate. However, a glance at prenatal mortality indicates that males are more vulnerable even in this equally sheltered environment. Of the 6,000 embryos and fetuses in the collection at the Carnegie Institution of Washington, the ratio was 107.9 males to 100 females (Landreth, 1958).

The U.S. Public Health figures of 1959 reveal an infant mortality among the U.S. white population of 26.3 males to 20.0 females per 1000 births, while Ratcliff is cited as indicating that there were 160 male embryos lost through miscarriage compared to every 100 females (Hurlock, 1953). Winchester (1961) makes note of the fact that the ratio of boys to girls in multiple births is lower than for single births and becomes increasingly lower with increases in the number of multiple births. In the United States, the ratio of twins is 103.5 boys to each 100 girls; for triplets, it is 98 boys to each 100 girls; while, for quadruplets, it drops to 70 boys for each 100 girls. Furthermore, it is pointed out that in regions where poor nutrition, insufficient medical care, and crowded conditions occur, there is a relatively lower birth ratio of males to females in comparison to areas having a high standard of living.

Clearly, then, females are the constitutionally stronger sex and it is felt that this stronger constitution may be the result of the balancing effect of paired genes in the two X chromosomes of the female. In support of this theory, Landreth (1958) cites the fact that, along with a higher mortality rate at all age levels, males are more likely to have congenital deformities.

MUTATIONS

The appearance of mutations, which involve chemical changes in the genetic structure that are capable of being transmitted to future generations of offspring through the germ cells, is the only currently known method of genetic alteration. Although we are not aware of all the factors which may cause mutations, we do know that mutations are more likely to occur in the germ cells of older fathers and that high levels of radiation will contribute to the increased appearance of mutations in both sexes. The latter knowledge has been of utmost importance in world affairs since the development of the atomic bomb.

A mutation which received a great deal of prominence in the early 20th century because of the political ramifications resulting from its appearance was that of hemophelia in the offspring of Queen Victoria. Since inheritance lines in many royal families are traced through the male offspring, the sudden appearance of this mutation had serious repercussions in the royal families of Germany, Russia, and Spain. Edward, Queen Victoria's father, was 52 years old at the time of Victoria's birth and it is now conjectured that his chromosome was the site of the mutation (McKusick, 1965).

Although its mechanism of operation has not been understood until relatively recently, the importance of heredity has long been appreciated by man. The development of the electron microscope and of atomic reactors and accelerators is opening the immense field of biophysics to the geneticist and medical researcher. It is now considered theoretically possible that some day the biochemists and biophysicists may be able to replace a "bad" gene with a "good" gene by shifting a few bases in molecules of DNA (Cooley, 1963). A large number of diseases, as familiar as diabetes or as unfamiliar as phenylketonuria are suspected or known to have a genetic component. Cancer, although not a specific disease, is in all instances a manifestation of tissue malfunction. Since the thousands of sequences of the four bases of the DNA molecule constitute the code-script that controls the development and functioning of the cells of the body, it is theoretically possible that the secret to this dread malady and of other conditions having a genetic component may be unlocked with increased knowledge of the hereditary mechanisms.

CHAPTER II

PRENATAL MATERNAL INFLUENCES

With the maturation of the reproductive germ cells into the egg and sperms, as the case may be, the hereditary contribution of the parents to the potential offspring is completed. If no union is effected between the egg and a sperm, the egg disintegrates. However, fertilization of the egg by the penetration of its wall by a sperm marks the conception of a new offspring and from this moment the environment in which the individual grows and develops influences the extent of attainment of the hereditary contributions.

PRENATAL DEVELOPMENTAL PERIODS

When, in the course of its progress down the Fallopian tube from the ovary to the uterus, the egg is fertilized, the haploid number of chromosomes in the gametes (sperm and egg) combine to form a cell with 46 chromosomes and, in so doing, trigger off the processes that result in the development of a human individual. The wall of the zygote (fertilized ovum) becomes impermeable to additional sperms and mitotic cell division begins. It takes the fertilized ovum approximately a week to complete its journey down the Fallopian tube, during which time it is constantly undergoing mitotic division with its only nourishment being the material stored in the original egg.

By the time the zygote reaches the uterus, it has developed little burr-like tendrils on the outside and, with these, implants itself in the prepared wall of the uterus. Implantation usually occurs approximately 10 days after fertilization. During this time, the original single cell has divided into a global cluster of cells having separate inner and outer layers. Upon implantation, the outer layer of cells begins to develop into the accessory tissues which will protect and provide the means by which the individual will obtain nourishment from and eliminate waste products to the mother, while the inner layer continues to divide until it in turn forms a global cluster of three layers of cells. This period from conception until two weeks later when parasitic connections have been completed with the wall of the uterus is known as the germinal period.

The next six weeks, known as the period of the embryo, are remarkable for the rapid and marked changes that take place as, from a cluster of undifferentiated cells, there develops a miniature individual complete with all essential internal and external features, some not yet functional, encased in a protective world of its own making. During the early part of the six weeks, the external cell layer that was previously formed develops into the amniotic sac, the placenta, the umbilical cord, and the chorion. As the amniotic membrane enlarges, it becomes filled with the amniotic fluid which has a definite chemical make-up and a specific gravity of 1006-1081 (Feldman, 1920). Meanwhile, at the end of the developing umbilical cord, the inner layer of cells developed during the germinal period continues to divide until three layers of cells are formed; namely, the ectoderm, the mesoderm, and the endoderm. The ectoderm or outer layer, continues its development to differentiate into the epidermis of the skin, the nails, hair, parts of the teeth, the sensory cells, the skin glands, and the entire nervous system. The mesoderm, or middle layer, eventually forms the dermis, or inner layer of the skin, the skeletal and muscular structures, and the circulatory and excretory organs while the endoderm, or inner layer, differentiates to produce the lining of the digestive tract, the respiratory system, the liver, the salivary glands, and various glands of internal secretion.

Some concept of the phenomenal development and differentiation that takes place during the six week period of the embryo which marks the conversion of a pin-head sized mass of cells into a recognizable human individual even though its 1½ to 2 inches of length is comprised of an enormous head, a rounded, elongated trunk, very small arms and legs with elbow and knee joints, webbed fingers and toes, and, moreover, a vestigial tail, may be gained from Figure 5, which diagrams the relationship between the uterus, the membranes, and the embryo.

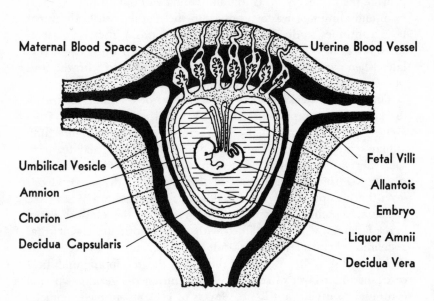

Figure 5.   Diagram representing the relationship between the uterus, the membranes, and the embryo during pregnancy. (From "The Onset and Early Development of Behavior" by L. Carmichael. In L. Carmichael (Ed.), **Manual of Child Psychology.** 2d. ed., New York: John Wiley & Sons, Inc., 1954. By permission of the publisher.)

Since the development of the placenta and the umbilical cord are completed early in the embryonic period, it is highly possible that the resultant increased food supply available to the organism may act as a stimulant to growth and development. It is, moreover, important to note that there is no direct connection between the fetal and maternal blood vessels and that food and oxygen for the embryo and waste products from the embryo must be filtered through a living membrane. There are also no neural connections between the mother and the fetus which rules out the possibility, as is sometimes believed, that the nervous condition of the mother will directly affect the child.

The period of the fetus, which extends from the end of the second month until birth, is one where development consists mainly of changes in the relative or actual size of the body parts rather than in the appearance of new parts. During the early part of this period there is a rapid increase in body length. As the rate of growth in this dimension declines, rapid increases in limb length occur. A sevenfold increase in trunk length and an eightfold increase in limb length alter the body proportions. The head, which was, at the end of the embryonic period, $\frac{1}{3}$ of the body length, becomes slightly less than $\frac{1}{4}$ and the trunk less than $\frac{1}{2}$ the total length, while the limbs are a little more than $\frac{1}{4}$ of the body length at the time of birth.

All the internal organs are well developed by the end of the third lunar month and, in some instances, begin to function at this time. The third lunar month also marks the appearance of short, threadlike prolongations of the nervous system that will later develop into the axons and dendrites of the neurons. So rapid is the development of these latter that within two months the complete number of neurons possessed by the mature adult are present although many of them are still in an immature state. Subsequent development of the nervous system involves extension of the axons and dendrites, modification of the synapses, and acquisition of myelin sheaths. By the end of the seventh lunar month, the fetus has reached the state of development which would make survival possible should birth occur at this time. This is referred to as the age of viability. However, the body is not completely formed until the end of the next month and chances of survival increase as the age of the fetus approaches that of a normal full term.

TERM OF PREGNANCY

Although the normal term of pregnancy is usually placed at 280 days, Needham (1931) has summarized the estimates of a number of investigators and found them to vary from 270 to 284 days while another survey (Landreth, 1958) indicates that ⅔ of all pregnancies terminate within 2 weeks, plus or minus, of 279 days. Although the opinion has been expressed that it may be possible to successfully rear premature infants who have passed less than 180 days in the mother's body, the average lower limit below which viability cannot be maintained is usually taken to be 180 days (Hess, 1922). However, the weight of the infant is also an important consideration in premature viability since survival is doubtful if the child is under 3 pounds at birth. Prematurity, in and of itself, has associated with it the provision of a suitable environment including the proper adjustment of oxygen supply, too much of which is now known to cause blindness (Landreth, 1958). At the postmaturity end of the scale, Ballantyne and Browne (1922) indicate that 334 days may be the longest legally considered period for the fetus to have remained inside the mother's body and still be delivered alive. There may, therefore, in the most extreme possible cases, be a range of 154 days during which viability can occur in the birth of human infants.

MULTIPLE BIRTHS

Sometimes, rather than the usual single egg, two eggs may be present in the Fallopian tubes and both of these may be fertilized by two different sperms. In this case, the development of both fertilized ova would proceed as if only one ovum were present except for the restrictions that the uterine cavity would have to be shared by the developing individuals as would the nourishment available from the mother. The space limitations would impose restrictions upon the size and activity of the two developing fetuses while the food and oxygen limitations would also affect size and activity. Twins produced from the fertilization of separate ova by separate sperms are called non-identical, or fraternal twins, and have no greater genetic similarity to each other than to their other brothers and sisters. Furthermore, they may be of either sex. They tend, however, to show greater similarity in acquired characteristics than do ordinary siblings because of the greater similarity in their experiences as they grow up together.

It is also possible that, instead of dividing and maintaining a cohesion between the two new cells during the first mitotic division, a fertilized ovum may divide so that no cohesion exists between the two new cells and these in turn continue to divide and develop independently into two separate individuals who have a common genetic background. Winchester (1961) cites a simple but dramatic experiment to illustrate this process. If a fertilized salamander egg is pinched in two along the line of demarcation between the cells after the first mitotic division, the two separated cells will continue to divide and differentiate until eventually each develops into a complete salamander. Human twins formed by this cleavage process are identical with respect to their genetic inheritance and are consequently always of the same sex. They also have identical hair-whorl patterns; the same color and pattern in the iris of the eyes; the same hair texture; and similarly shaped ears, lips and eyebrows. Physiologically, they have the same blood type, subtype and Rh factor and it has been found that skin grafts and kidney transplantations may be successfully made from one identical twin to another.

Approximately once in every four identical twin births, a phenomenon called mirror-imaging occurs. In this instance, the physical characteristics of one side of one twin's body are reflected in the opposite side of the other twin so that if one twin's hair spirals clockwise, the other s hair does so in a counterclockwise direction; one twin's heart and appendix are on the left side, the other twin's are on the right; dental irregularities appear on opposite sides while opposing eyes are dominant. Since one's impression of one's personal appearance is gained from observation of one's image in a mirror, it is easy to believe stories of mirror-image twins talking to their reflection in an unexpected mirror in the belief that it is their mirror-image twin (Hicks, 1963).

Multiple human births may also occur in threes, fours, fives, and even sixes, with the likelihood of occurrence of twin births being once in approximately 85 births; triplets, once in 7,225 births; quadruplets, once in every 614,125 births; and quintuplets, once in every 52,200,625 births (Hurlock, 1953). There have been approximately 40 recorded cases of the birth of quintuplets with the Dionne quintuplets, who are identical, being the first set to survive to adulthood. The Diligenti quintuplets of Argentina were the second group to survive and are a fraternal set being composed of two boys and three girls. Of the four authenticated cases of the birth of sextuplets, there has been no instance of even temporary survival proven for any one of the infants (Hicks, 1963).

From the preceeding discussion, it is obvious that both fraternal and identical twins may be found in all categories of multiple births. With triplets, there can be three different combinations; namely, 1) A single egg fertilized by a single sperm divides and one of the resulting two eggs divides again. This results in identical triplets. 2) Two separate sperms fertilize two separate eggs of which one divides to form twins. This results in two identical twins and one fraternal twin. 3) Three separate eggs are fertilized by three separate sperms resulting in fraternal triplets. Similarly, there can be five different combinations with quadruplets and seven with quintuplets.

The age of the mother seems to have some influence on the likelihood of the occurrence of multiple births. Older women are more likely to have twins than are younger women. A woman of 40 is three or four times as likely to have twins as a woman 20 years old with the maximal twin frequency occurring when the mother is in her 37th year. The age of the father has no effect on the twin rate. Furthermore, the tendency towards identical multiple births may be inherited from either parent whereas the tendency towards fraternal twins is carried principally by the female. There are some remarkable family histories such as those of a Sicilian woman who produced 11 sets of fraternal twins in as many years, and an Australian woman who is reported to have borne 69 children including 4 sets of quadruplets, 7 sets of triplets, and 16 sets of twins (Hicks, 1963).

PRENATAL MATERNAL INFLUENCES

Even within the mother's body, survival is beset with numerous problems. During the period of the ovum, the yolk must have enough nourishment to enable the zygote to complete its journey down the Fallopian tubes to the uterus or it will die. If the uterus has not been properly prepared to receive the ovum, implantation cannot occur and the fertilized egg disintegrates from lack of nourishment (Hurlock, 1953). Although the living membrane in the placenta acts as a filter through which food and oxygen pass to reach the developing individual, it is also permeable to alcohol, nicotine, drugs, and some viruses and bacteria. If the mother's diet is insufficient to meet the demands of the developing fetus, the latter exerts a parasitic effect in various ways, for example, the robbing of the mother's teeth of calcium. Certain glandular conditions of the mother may indirectly affect the fetus as hormonal secretions filter through the placenta. Thus violent emotional states of the mother may be reflected in unusual activity of the fetus. The embryo seems to be particularly susceptible to maternal conditions, as this first six weeks after implantation is the period of rapid differentiation of the various organs of the body and as such is the most crucial and vulnerable period in an organ's development.

NUTRITION

The nutritional adequacy of the expectant mother's diet seems to have a very definite effect upon the condition of the newborn infant, its size, and the length of its term. A study made by Burke et al. (1943) reports that where the mother's diet was excellent, 95 percent of the children were born in excellent condition whereas in instances where the mother's diet was poor, only 8 percent of the infants were in excellent condition. Furthermore, a positive correlation of .80 was found between the length of the infant and the protein intake of the mother.

Since proteins are necessary for human growth and are obtainable in quantity and quality only in the more expensive foods such as meats and fishes, it may be assumed that they would tend to be in inadequate supply among low income groups and, as such, affect the condition of the infants in these groups. This surmise tends to be confirmed by the results of a study by Baird (1945) of the relationship between prematurity and the income of the family, with observations indicating that the percentage of prematurity was twice as high in the lower income groups of Scotland than it was among those groups of higher status, both economic and social.

That prematurity and the condition of the child is not entirely based upon economic status, however, is indicated by Baird's findings that the groups in the higher social classifications, who may be considered to be better educated even though they do not have the monetary advantage of being in the higher economic groups, still tended to maintain a high protein diet for the mother during the term of pregnancy and the period during which the child was being breast fed. These families, with their better understanding of the nutritional demands made upon the mother at this time, obviously make the necessary arrangements to supply the greater protein needs required by the mother (Landreth, 1958).

Moral considerations prevent us from conducting experimental studies with human beings in which there is a possibility of damage or injury to the individuals taking part in such a study. Consequently, there have been no experimental studies of the relationship between maternal dietary deficiencies and deformities in children. However, it may be assumed that such a relationship exists on the basis of a study where a diet deficient in a nutrient required for adequate protein synthesis was fed to pregnant rats after various numbers of days of normal feeding following breeding. When the deficient diet was fed to the pregnant rats starting 9 days after breeding until birth of the offspring, all the litters were stillborn. The feeding of the deficient diet from 11 days after breeding until birth resulted in 95 percent of the young being littered alive but they exhibited multiple congenital deformities. One hundred percent of the young were littered live with only mild congenital abnormalities when the deficient diet was started 12 to 13 days after breeding, whereas, after 15 days of normal feeding, the change to the deficient diet seemed to have no effect as normal litters were produced (Nelson et al., 1952).

It is highly unlikely that even in the most extreme economic circumstances one would meet the stringent conditions of diet that can be imposed in laboratory experiments. However, such experiments, together with the observations of maternal diet and condition of human offspring, do point up the necessity of maintenance of a nutritionally adequate diet for the expectant and nursing mother.

MATERNAL INFECTIONS

It has been found that when rubella, or German measles, is contracted in the first month of pregnancy, the expectant mother has a 50-50 chance of delivering a defective child. Even in the second or third month contraction of the disease presents an 8 percent chance of delivery of a deformed child, with the defects including congenital deafness, cataracts, abnormal heart formation and mental retardation. As the early differentiation of the organs most affected by the disease takes place during this time, it would appear that these organs tend to pass through a critical period in development in which they are most susceptible to certain environmental influences. Since the possibility of malformation of the child is very great for an expectant mother who contracts rubella, special effort should be made to avoid all contacts with the disease during pregnancy.

As well as causing deformities during early pregnancy, some maternal infections may be transmitted to the unborn child and result in its birth with the condition or its death. Some of the infections that may result in the death of the infant are influenza, smallpox, typhoid fever, chicken pox, measles, and syphilis, with the latter disease also presenting the alternatives of blindness or other abnormalities, as well as premature and stillbirths. Other maternal infections which, through the condition of the mother, will usually result in the death of the unborn child are cholera, erysipelas, and malaria.

DRUGS

Such a period of susceptibility to environmental influences is also shown in other organ development with a very highly publicized recent instance being that of the tranquilizing drug, thalidomide. It was found that a high incidence of malformed births occurred when the drug was taken by an expectant mother in the early stages of her pregnancy, with the most obvious defects being congenital deformities such as paddle appendages or lack of limb development as well as heart and other internal organ deformities. In West Germany, where the drug was easily available from 1957 to 1962, an estimated 5,000 malformed births were attributed to the drug with about 2,000 of these babies dying as a result of their deformities. In the United States, however, later release and more stringent controls of the drug resulted in only 14 cases of gross deformities of newborn babies directly traceable to thalidomide. The publicity surrounding the discovery of the deforming effects of thalidomide resulted in its withdrawal from the market and pointed up the dangers associated with the administration of drugs to pregnant women.

Other drugs that have been found to have malforming and injurious effects have among their number quinine, the excessive use of which may result in deafness in the newborn child. Alcohol, consumed in excessive amounts by the mother during early pregnancy, may result in death or malformation, while nicotine has been found to have the same stimulating and depressant effects on the child that it does on the mother but to a larger magnitude as the same amount of nicotine is available to the smaller body area of the fetus. If the mother is engaged in industrial work involving lead or arsenic fumes, these substances will filter through the placenta to the fetus with the severity of the effects being dependent upon the amount inhaled by the mother. Narcotic drug consumption, such as opium or morphine, by the mother may result in the child entering the world as an addict, depending again on the amount of consumption by the mother.

RH INCOMPATIBILITY

An intra-uterine problem that may cause complications during pregnancy is the incompatibility of Rh blood types between the mother and her developing child. Although, as previously mentioned, there is no direct exchange of blood between the mother and her child, there may, toward the end of the pregnancy when the weight and the movements of the fetus cause some capillary breakage in the placenta, be some seepage of blood from the fetus to the mother. In instances where an Rh negative mother is carrying her first Rh positive child, this seepage results in the production of antibodies in the mother's blood for it has no Rh factor and her body therefore treats the Rh factor in the blood that has entered her system from the child as a noxious substance. Since this seepage usually occurs towards the end of pregnancy and it takes some time for the mother to develop antibodies to the Rh factor, this process usually has no effect upon the first Rh positive child born to the Rh negative mother. However, the sensitization that has been produced in the mother may have been great enough to develop a titre of antibodies that may be sufficiently high to affect the blood cells of the embryos of any future Rh positive pregnancies. In this instance, the second, or any subsequent, Rh positive child will be born with erythroblastosis fetalis, a condition which is characterized by immature, nucleated red blood cells that are inefficient carriers of oxygen, and with anemia and jaundice (Winchester, 1961).

Since 85 percent of the population has Rh positive blood and the foregoing situation only occurs in instances when marriage involves an Rh positive man and an Rh negative woman—the gene for the Rh factor is dominant—some indication is given as to the likelihood of Rh incompatability resulting from a marriage. Surveys indicate that approximately 12 percent of marriages involve Rh positive males and Rh negative females. Of the total number of children of these marriages, a study in England found that one child in every 23 had erythroblastosis. However, this total included first born positive children as well as all Rh negative children so that, while the overall chance appears low, it masks the truth with respect to subsequent Rh positive children born to Rh negative mothers. Here the danger is very great and a physician can be readily alerted to possible incompatability, if the mother has been found to be Rh negative, by testing blood samples from the father and all previous children or by the previous births of children with erythroblastosis. In the event of the live birth of a child with erythroblastosis, the child may be saved by draining off some of the damaged blood and replacing it with transfusions of compatible Rh positive blood immediately after birth and during the first few subsequent days (Winchester, 1961). The previously high mortality rate of 45 percent for live births with erythroblastosis has now been reduced to 5 percent by this exchange transfusion of blood (The National Foundation—March of Dimes).

POSITION OF FETUS

Another factor in the intra-uterine environment of the fetus that affects its development is its position in the uterus. It has been found that pressure on the tips of the bones stimulates ossification of the bone. However, the fetus must relax in order to accommodate to its cramped quarters in the uterus so that, in instances of excessive relaxation of the hip ligaments, it is possible that the lack of pressure will result in the birth of a child with a congenital cartilaginous dislocated hip. Such a defect may be remedied by medical treatment after birth (Landreth, 1958).

Although mal-development of the limb bud may also be the cause, it is possible that clubfoot, which occurs in 1 out of approximately 250 live births, may be due to the position of the child in the uterus. Since correction involves the stretching of muscles and ligaments and the realignment of bones, treatment must begin early and is usually prolonged as the condition tends to recur (The National Foundation—March of Dimes). In instances of multiple births, the cramped quarters and the more limited food supply available to each developing child tend to restrict motility and size of the infants and are more likely to produce deformities of the cartilaginous tissue.

Experiments with animals tend to indicate that cleft lip and palate may also be partially attributable to the position of the embryo or the blood supply in the uterus as well as having genetic components. Although a cleft palate will also occur in 70 percent of the 1 in approximately every 1,000 white births with a cleft lip, the two conditions are not genetically related, with cleft palate having an incidence of about 1 in every 2,500 babies (The National Foundation—March of Dimes). Investigations of the relationship of these conditions with regard to paternal age indicates that the risk of producing a child with cleft lip and cleft palate is increased in older parents (Woolf, 1963). Today many operative techniques are available for repairing these defects. Cleft lip, or more commonly, harelip, is repairable during the first few weeks after birth and cleft palate before the child is 14 months old in the majority of cases.

AGE OF PARENTS

Parental age would seem to have a very decided effect in instances where chromosomal changes or errors are responsible for mutations, as previously mentioned with regard to hemophelia in Queen Victoria's offspring, and for abnormalities such as mongolism where all individuals have chromosomal error; namely, 47 chromosomes or the equivalent instead of the normal complement of 46 chromosomes. In all instances of chromosomal error, the cause can, of course, be either hereditary or environmental, or both. However, the high incidence of mongolism, an average expectation of about

1 child in every 50 births for women 45 years and over, in contrast with the expectancy of about 1 child in 2,000 births for women of 25 years of age, certainly indicates that the environmental factor, in this case, age, plays a very important role. Since mongolism has an occurrence of 1 in 600 for all ages it would seem the incidence may also be higher at the younger age limits. Certainly, statistics for all birth defects show that mothers under 18 years and over 40 years of age have a higher proportion of children with birth defects than those between the ages of 18 and 40 years (The National Foundation—March of Dimes).

HORMONE DEFICIENCIES

Since women under 18 years of age are probably still undergoing physiological adjustments to the increased estrogen production that marks biological maturity and women over 40 years are making physiological adjustments to decreased estrogen production, it is highly likely that hormonal imbalance is an adjunct of the age relationship to birth defects. It has been found that the mothers of mongoloid children have tended to have a history of threatened abortions, impaired hormone regulation, menstrual irregularities, ovarian abnormalities, menopausal symptoms, or difficulties in becoming pregnant. It is also believed that a deficiency of maternal thyroxine in the early development of the embryo or of iodine in the later stages of pregnancy may be the cause of cretinism which, although it only occurs in approximately 2 children in every 10,000 births, has, as does mongolism, no known cure (Landreth, 1958).

Taking as a definition of a serious birth defect one that either results in a physical or mental handicap, causes disfigurement, shortens life, or is fatal, there is, in this country, a proportion of 1 baby in every 16 born with a serious birth defect. In order to help insure a healthy baby, the National Foundation—March of Dimes recommends that prospective parents give consideration to the following:

1. There is danger in marrying a close relative, as such a marriage increases the risk of compounding the errors in heredity.
2. A newly married couple should select a family physician who should be informed of any family history of defects and should complete thorough medical examinations of both parties. In

the event of pregnancy, it is important that both parents realize the necessity of proper prenatal care to avoid premature births and also the necessity of being alerted to possible complications such as Rh incompatability.

3. Every mother should be sure to tell her doctor if she thinks she is pregnant and should take only the medicines he prescribes.

4. Since there is a correlation between certain virus diseases and birth defects, the pregnant mother should make a special effort to avoid contact with such diseases. Moreover, as severe damage can occur from rubella even in the early weeks after conception before the woman realizes she is pregnant, it would probably be safer for future children if all females, 12 years of age and under, contracted the disease, as it is a relatively light illness of short duration during childhood and one attack provides an individual with lifetime immunity. However, advances in vaccine development may soon provide a much more convenient means of immunity.

5. Abdominal x-rays should be avoided during the early weeks of pregnancy, except in emergency.

6. As studies show there is an inverse relationship between the number of cigarettes a mother smokes and the weight of her newborn child, excessive smoking should be avoided during pregnancy.

7. The high correlation between birth defects and the age of the mother would indicate the desirability of planning for parenthood between the ages of 18 and 40 years.

8. Since diet affects growth, proper eating habits acquired early in a girl's life will be conducive not only to her own good health but also to that of her prospective children.

CHAPTER III

DIFFERENTIATION AND INTEGRATION OF THE SENSORY-MOTOR SYSTEM

With the fusion of the ovum and sperm, the destiny of the new individual becomes a product of the genetic information stored in the newly united protoplasm and the environment in which it develops. Cell division involving both differentiation into new structures and increase in mass of existing structure takes place immediately. During embryonic development in particular, it is vital that these processes balance each other in order to supply both the diverse types of cells required for the efficient functioning of a multi-celled organism and for maintenance of the inherited integrity of the fertilized ovum for future transmission to offspring. There must be orderly cell division, differentiation, unification, and integration to the end that the structuring and functioning of the organism can be classified phylogenetically as human.

The major mechanism affecting these processes is not clearly understood. It may be that balance in development is maintained by chromosomal DNA (Waddington, 1962) in combination with the non-chromosomal DNA found in mitochondria (Sager, 1965). So complex is the process of organized differentiation that DNA, despite its remarkable properties cannot be the sole determinant. Others may be spatial cytoplasmic distribution with respect to the polarity of the cell (Waddington, 1962), the pressure exerted on a cell by the surrounding structures, and the metabolic status of the cell (Landreth, 1958). The interactions of chemicals in the cell membranes may be a factor both in cell differentiation and in the unification of similar cells into multi-celled structures (Waddington, 1962). Unfortunately, little is known about these phenomena in general although new instruments and new techniques such as the electron microscope and radiation analysis are assisting greatly in advancing knowledge.

The development of bones and muscles appears to be somewhat less complex with respect to the integration processes than does that of the nervous system. Differentiation of all of these structures would seem, in terms of our present knowledge, to be adequately covered by the determinants previously discussed. Integration of the function of the bones and muscles and to some extent that of the nerves may be explained by the position and timing at which differentiation occurs in the developing limb bud (Waddington, 1962) as well as by interactions of chemicals in the cell membranes. However, in dealing with the interaction of the nervous system, the mechanisms whereby each sensory and motor nerve achieves its proper terminal ending would seem to be more numerous, if not any more complex than those already mentioned, because of the variety both in end organs and in the specificity of their function. Probably the embryonic processes for the inherent patterning of the neuronal linkages, as well as the grosser phases of neurogenesis, are the same as those for the other organ systems (Sperry, 1951). Since the nervous system is the mechanism by which the organism is made aware of its external and internal environment and whereby it transmits its reactions to such stimuli, the functional integration of this system has been subjected to a great deal of investigation. Some of these studies will be of interest here.

SENSORY NEURON DEVELOPMENT

Since new fibers frequently must traverse considerable distances to reach their terminal endings, researchers have been intrigued by the fact that each fiber follows a specific path. It has been found that growth takes place only when the nerve fiber is in contact with a supporting surface and never just in a homogeneous media (Harrison, 1914). However, various structures, even those as small as delicate interfacial films or even ultramicroscopic particles of interstitial fluid will deflect or channel the fine filamentous pseudopodia of the advancing nerve fiber tips (Weiss, 1941a). This indicates the importance of mechanical factors in the guidance of growing nerves toward their destination.

But a considerable body of evidence has been accumulated to suggest that chemical forces are even more important in impelling a nerve in a specific direction. Nerve generation studies, especially on amphibians, have supplied the major portion of our knowledge in this area. Piatt (1942), for example, observed that retarded invasion of nerves into a previously innervated area proceeded in a normal fashion. He grafted limbs, which had grown on parabiotic salamander twins to an advanced stage of development in the complete absence of innervation, in place of the corresponding limbs on the otherwise normal twin counterpart. The resultant nerve pattern formed by the invasion of the host nerves into the developed limbs that had not previously been innervated was found to be remarkably normal. Many features of the process, such as the entrances of the nerves into their muscles at their customary points, the penetration of the cartilage masses by the nerves, and the tunnelling of the ulnar nerve through the belly of the ulno-carpal muscle instead of coursing around it, indicate the vitality of the process and suggest that the different nerve fibers are prone to grow preferentially along pathways with specific chemical properties.

Other investigators have noted that growing nerves show a marked tendency to deviate from normal pathways in order to arrive at and make connection with displaced organ tissue. In some instances nerves seem to be able to induce the appropriate end organs to develop at their terminal points. The theory has been advanced that this is brought about by a high degree of biochemical specificity (Speidel, 1946; Olmsted, 1931; Bailey, 1937). A somewhat lesser degree of biochemical specificity is exhibited by the nerve fibers of the general cutaneous system, as these terminate freely without inducing any specialized endings (Speidel, 1948). Occasionally nerve fibers can be forced to form atypical terminations but at no time do adrenergic fibers form functional connections with cholinergic endings or vice versa. Sensory nerve fibers are also unable to form transmissive junctions with motor nerve fibers (Langley and Anderson, 1904; Weiss and Edds, 1945).

Further support to theories of neuronal biochemical specificity is lent by studies where atypical connections have been induced by surgery. Following surgical rotation of the eye of the frog combined with severence of the spinal cord, Sperry (1942, 1943, 1944) made a histological examination of the optic axons at the point of regeneration and found that, while the axons became thoroughly disarranged during the course of regeneration, the reassociation of the various fibers during regeneration was not achieved in a random manner, since there was a persistant systematic reversal of the visuomotor reactions directly correlated with the rotated position of the retina after recovery.

Further studies by Sperry and colleagues show clearly that this specificity is present in the very early stages of the development of the organism and cannot be changed by surgical rearrangement. Transplantation of skin flaps with their original innervation intact across the midline of the metamorphosing tadpole before it has had any experience with localizing responses results, in the adult frog upon stimulation of the displaced flaps, in wiping reactions to the original site of the skin flaps (Sperry, 1951). In another study, the dorsal roots of the hind limb nerves of the tadpole are cross-connected with those on the opposite side of the cord (Figure 6). Later, the adult frog exhibits characteristic reflex reactions in the opposite leg while the foot being stimulated remains motionless (Sperry, 1951).

Where the same operation is performed on adult frogs the proprioceptive reflex relations are restored in a selective manner. Following surgical displacement of the dorsal roots in the adult frog, the reaction of the contralateral limb is conditioned by the position of the stimulated limb. For example, if the stimulated right foot is extended, a stimulus applied to this foot will result in flexion of the left leg while, if the stimulated right foot is in a position of flexion, the stimulus will result in extension of the left leg. This reaction will take place, or be attempted, as a result of stimulation regardless of the position of the limb contralateral to the limb being stimulated. As a check on these results, Sperry (1951) observed

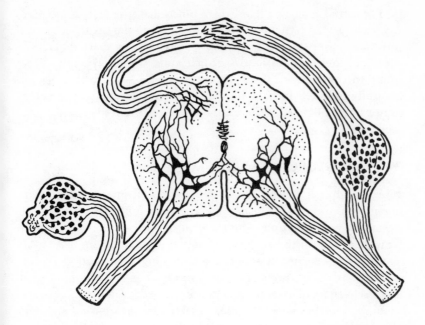

Figure 6.   Contralateral cross union of dorsal roots. When the dorsal roots of the hind-limb nerves are crossed in the manner indicated, the regenerating sensory root fibers establish functional relations with the spinal centers of the contralateral limb similar to those that they establish with the ipsilateral limb centers. This selective formation of the central reflex connections cannot be attributed either to mechanical guidance or to functional adjustment. (From "Mechanisms of Neural Maturation" by R. W. Sperry. In S. S. Stevens (Ed.), **Handbook of Experimental Psychology.** New York: John Wiley & Sons, Inc., 1951. By permission of the publisher.)

similar influences of the leg's posture upon its own responses after the ipsilateral regeneration of surgically severed dorsal roots.

These studies suggest that, where functional specificity is required, in such sensory systems as the visual, vestibular, cutaneous, and proprioceptive, the end organ tissue undergoes primary differentiation and then induces local specificity into whatever sensory fibers come in contact with them. In other sensory systems, specificity is neurally induced. In both instances, patterns formed at the neural centers remain fixed despite any subsequent forced atypical connections.

MOTOR NEURON DEVELOPMENT

Although it is possible that a similar mechanism of selective axon outgrowth to their proper peripheral connections may operate with regard to motor neurons, studies seem to indicate that, in amphibians, the outgrowth and termination of spinal motor neurons is entirely non-selective in both development and regeneration (Weiss, 1937; Piatt, 1940). Saunders (1947) has expressed the opinion that some selectivity of axon termination is assured, under normal conditions, by the chronological order in which the neurons differentiate and send forth their axons and by the proximo-distal order in which the limb segments develop. Weiss (1936, 1941b) on the other hand, maintains that a considerable amount of freedom remains to the motor neurons invading any limb segment since the proper muscular coordination is achieved even with highly random outgrowth and termination in the periphery. The resultant implication that the central connections must be adjusted secondarily to suit the peripheral innervation is strengthened by the observation that the timing of the central discharge becomes adapted to the new terminals even when divided motor axons are forced to regenerate into entirely foreign muscles.

Weiss (1941b) also noted that the adaptation of the timing of the central discharge was not achieved by a learning process for, even when the limbs of amphibians are transplanted to the contralateral side and reversed in such a way that the resultant movement of the limbs tends to push the animal backward when it attemps to go forward and vice versa, the individual movement patterning of the limbs persists despite its obvious malfunctioning. When similar limb transplants are made in prefunctional stages of the amphibian's development, similar effects are obtained indicating that these relations are patterned initially through developmental forces and not through any kind of functional adjustment. Additional studies showed that these motor patterns developed in the same systematic way in the absence of sensory innervation and, furthermore, they persisted in the animal after decerebration and cord transection down to the levels of the cord just rostral to the limb segments (Weiss, 1937c). These results ruled out the possibility that learning or any type of functional adaptation may have produced specificity in the patterning of the peripheral neuro-muscular relations.

There must be some sort of central discrimination of motor neurons according to the muscles they innervate because the timing of the central discharges is always adjusted on this basis. Since Weiss only disturbed the end-organ, or peripheral, connections in his experiments, he concluded that the motor neurons possess some constitutional, presumably biochemical, specificity induced in them by their muscles. It follows, then, that each muscle must have biochemical properties of its own. This explanation would also serve to account for the differentiation of the limb musculature during its morphogenetic development. If one accepts the hypothesis that biochemical muscular specificity induces biochemical specificity in motor neurons then it becomes possible to explain the relationship between peripheral motor connections and the sensory and central nervous systems in terms of the general chemoaffinity theory of synaptic patternings (Sperry, 1951).

Central synaptic connections are assumed, under the connectionist theory, to be originally established on a selective chemoaffinity basis depending upon the biochemical specificity of the motor neurons which in turn has previously been induced by the specificity of the terminal muscle. Once the biochemical specificity of the motor neurons has been established, it is assumed that the sensory and association neurons form their synaptic connections among the motor neurons in a selective manner on the basis of this biochemical specificity. In cases where motor axons regenerate into foreign muscles, the new muscles are believed to induce a biochemical change in the motor neurons.

In the light of the foregoing discussion, it is obvious that definite information is still lacking as to the precise developmental organization of the entire sensory-neuro-motor mechanism. However, it is possible to make surmises with respect to some of the reflex circuits. Myotatic reflexes have been found to be mediated by a two-neuron arc comprised of the proprioceptive sensory and the primary motor neurons (Lloyd, 1946). If the theories discussed above apply to the acquisition of specificity and central connections in such a two-neuron arc, then the motor neuron forms its peripheral connections with the muscle fiber, attains its induced biochemical specificity, after which it develops wide-spreading dendrites in the spinal cord. In the meantime, the sensory neuron has attained its end-organ relations and has sent its central root fibers into the cord in ascending and descending branches. These branches later send off numerous collaterals into the neuropil with some of them making direct contact with the cell body and dendrites of the motor neuron. When forming synaptic connections, the afferent sensory fibers from each muscle exhibit a special affinity for those motor neurons biochemically specified by the same muscle. They also show some degree of affinity for the motor neurons of the most closely related muscles. Such simplicity of interneuronal connections as the two-neuron arc are rare, however, and it is highly probable that the same proprioceptive root fibers may form connections on a different basis on other levels of the cord. So complex is the problem of sensory-motor innervation and so painstaking the research in the area that, although the concept of reciprocal innervation was advanced by Sherrington in 1906 to account for the action of the agonists and antagonists in muscular action, we are still not sure of the neural basis of reciprocal innervation (Eccles, 1965; Wilson, 1966).

MUSCLE STRUCTURE AND INNERVATION

Since it has been found that the innervation ratio of muscle fibers to each neuron varies from one gross muscle to another and also, to a lesser extent, within each gross muscle, a quick review of the structure of the muscle is appropriate here. A gross muscle is made up of numerous muscle fibers separated from each other and into various sized bundles by connective tissue. The smallest unit, the muscle fiber, varies greatly in length and diameter among muscles but is relatively consistent within each gross muscle. In the adult human being, striated muscle fibers vary from 1 mm. in the stapedius muscle to 34 cm. in the startorious muscle with the smaller fibers generally being associated with finer movements. Diameter sizes, ranging from 10 to 150 microns, also show this type of distinctive association with movement, for the greater diameters are found in the larger muscles such as the gluteus maximus (Harrison, 1962).

The connective tissue surrounding each muscle fiber is called the endomysium while the connective tissue surrounding the small bundles, or fasciculi, in which the muscle fibers are arranged parallel to each other is called the perimysium. The fasciculi, also called bundles of the first order, or primary bundles, contain from 10 to 300 muscle fibers depending upon the type of muscle. These primary bundles are, in turn, arranged in parallel with several other primary bundles to form bundles of the second order. This structural arrangement is followed until the final bundle consists of the entire gross muscle itself which is covered with connective tissue called the epimysium. This abundance of connective tissue is important in the structure of the muscle and it serves as the harness against which the force of contraction of the muscle is directed. Various arrangements of the connective tissue, therefore, will result in diversification of movement.

Diversification in the contractive force of the gross muscle is mediated through the "motor unit"—the term given to the functional unit of muscular contraction comprised of the motor neuron and the muscle fibers activated by that neuron (Liddell and Sherrington, 1925). For the eye muscles, it has been found that approximately 5 to 8 muscle fibers are innervated by one motor nerve fiber. Similarly, approximately 25 muscle fibers have been found to be innervated by one motor nerve fiber for the platysma muscle; approximately 95 muscle fibers to one motor nerve fiber for the first lumbrical muscle; approximately 609 muscle fibers to one motor nerve fiber for the tibialis anterior muscle; and approximately 1,775 muscle fibers to one motor nerve fiber for the medial head of the gastrocnemius muscle. Innervation of the muscles indicates fewer muscle fibers per motor nerve fiber in the motor units mediating finer movements than in the motor units mediating gross movements. The muscle fibers of a motor unit are confined to an oval or circular area which is only a small fraction of the total cross section of the muscle and the territory encompassed by the motor unit does not seem to vary with the degree of development of the muscle. Furthermore, the territories encompassed by separate motor units overlap one another. Of a maximum of six units that have been found to overlap, two or three of the motor units have been found to overlap each other entirely so that their muscle fibers are assembled within the same region of the cross section of the gross muscle (Harrison, 1962).

After observing the reactions of the vastocrureus muscle in the decerebrate cat, Liddell and Sherrington (1925) concluded that the motor unit acted in an all-or-none fashion when its motor nerve was stimulated. The motor units, however, have gradient thresholds so that some motor nerves require minimal stimulation to trigger off the firing that causes muscular contraction whereas others do not fire until stronger stimulation triggers off the motor unit when stronger contractions are required. The strength of muscular contraction, then, is determined by the frequency and the number of motor units firing with a greater number of units being involved in a stronger contraction. However, the synchronous use of all the motor units in a gross muscle occurs very rarely, if at all. It appears that an exceptionally strong emotional stimulus would be necessary to trigger off the synchronous firing of all motor units. That such instances do occur is illustrated by stories of feats of exceptional strength under unusually strong emotional stimuli.

MYELINIZATION

The sheathing of the nerves with myelin is the final stage in their morphological development. The general correlation that has been found between the order in which nerves become functional and the order of the appearance of stainable myelin tends to suggest that there may be a relationship which is, however, not simple and tends to be of a reciprocal nature. Central nervous tracts become myelinated in a definite sequence which shows a considerable constancy in all the mammals and which tends to roughly follow the order in which tracts are developed phylogenetically. While the absence of function does not prevent the laying down of or decrease the ultimate degree of myelin (Romanes, 1947), it has been found that the laying down of myelin is stimulated and accelerated by function (Langworthy, 1933). Although Langworthy has shown that fairly complex activity can be carried out prior to myelinization, functions, in general, have been found to show a considerable improvement in speed, precision, steadiness, and strength coincident with the laying down of myelin. It would appear, then, that myelinization and the order of its appearance is an inherently determined process capable of proceeding in the absence of function in the usual sense but is also a process which is stimulated and accelerated by the presence of function.

This reciprocal mechanism which results in an acceleration in the laying down of myelin with increased function and in improved function as a result of increased myelinization is only effective within the limits of myelinization set down within the genetic inheritance of the individual. During the period of development of myelinization, the interrelationship of the myelinization–function process makes it difficult to assess the extent to which improved motor development is due to this process or to other maturational processes that may be going on simultaneously. However, the degree to which myelinization has been completed offers an excellent method of assessing the degree of maturation of the nervous system and, as such, is an indicator of the order and the degree to which various parts of the system become functional.

CHAPTER IV

PRENATAL DEVELOPMENT

Moral considerations and principles prevent us from conducting experimental studies in human embryology. Our limited knowledge of human prenatal development comes from premature fetuses that have not survived or those which have been surgically removed from the mother for medical reasons and have had no chance of survival. In these instances, it is obvious that behavior, if it can be elicited, will occur under a failing oxygen and food supply as well as under environmental conditions differing from the constant temperature, composition, and comparatively stimulus-free environment within the uterus. However, it has been found that there are stages in the morphological development of fish, amphibians, reptiles, birds, and infrahuman mammals which are similar to those in man so that it is possible to draw some inferences from studies of these creatures to augment and provide clues to the development of human behavior.

PRENATAL DEVELOPMENT IN INFRAHUMANS

As early as 1885, Preyer studied the development of trout (Coghill and Legner, 1937). A few days after fertilization of the egg he liberated the tiny fish from their coverings and continued at successive periods to do so with others of the organisms. He noted that movements became more and more regular and specific and increased in strength with age. After disappearance of the yolk sac definite changes in behavior were observed.

Exhaustive work has been done by Coghill (1929) in tracing the motor development of the salamander amblystoma. This investigator was the first to chart the relationship between detailed growth of the nervous system and the consequent alterations which occurred in behavior. A study of the neural structures in association with stages of development of the "S" or swimming reaction in the salamander, for example, showed that certain structures of the nervous system made possible specific types of behavior. The "S" reaction is clearly seen in the swimming of the lower vertebrates but is obscure in the locomotion of four legged mammals and even more so in the biped locomotion of human beings. However, Coghill believes this fundamental pattern may be a significant stage in the behavioral development of all higher organisms. He cites as evidence supporting his theory that when both sets of limbs first appear in the metamorphosing amphibian they move only with the trunk in swimming. Gradually the front legs achieve independence of action from the larger trunk movements and this is followed in turn by independence of limb action of the hind legs. The cephalocaudal progression of development of independent limb action repeats the cephalocaudal progression of trunk movements seen in the "S" reaction. Eventually the alternate positioning of the limbs in walking synchronizes with a reduced "S" reaction of the trunk during locomotion. Thus the "S" reaction is seen as a phylogenetic feature in the development of all vertebrates.

Some supporting evidence for the primacy of the "S" reaction may be found in the marsupials who give birth to their young in a condition equivalent to that of a very immature fetus in comparison with mammals. The fetal kangaroo and opossum travel directly from the vulva to the maternal pouch without any aid from the mother. Only the arms which are strongly developed are used to propel the body with the lower trunk merely trailing during the journey. This type of overhand swimming motion is reminiscent of the "S" reaction of the larval salamander.

This "S" type of reaction is not evident in the fetuses of four legged mammals such as the guinea pig which have their limbs fully formed before the occurrence of the first behavioral responses or reflexes. A very definite progression of stages in development can be traced, however. Bridgman and Carmichael (1935) found that myogenic responses could be elicited in the fetal guinea pig from certain muscles prior to the onset of behavior. "True" behavior, defined by these investigators as the responses resulting from stimulation, was next in order of appearance. These true behavior responses were sufficiently different in character from the earlier myogenic contractions to indicate that stimulation had induced a neural discharge to trigger off the muscular contraction. The first active responses of the fetal guinea pig were found to involve movements of the head caused by contraction of the neck muscles and movements of the four legs. They concluded that these earliest responses might advantageously be described as reflexes because of their simple and specific nature. They did not identify a gradual progressive individuation of specific responses out of a total pattern but rather identified the specific responses as primary.

Coronios (1933) made extensive studies on the fetal development of the cat. He formulated seven generalizations which typify the course of fetal development in infrahuman organisms.

1. Before birth, there is a rapid, progressive, and continuous development in the behavior of the fetus of the cat.
2. The development of behavior progresses from a diffuse, massive, variable, relatively unorganized state to a condition where many of the reactions are more regular in their appearance, less variable, better organized, and relatively individualized.
3. In the early stages of prenatal development the behavior appears to be progressing along a cephalocaudal course.
4. The development of the sensitivity of the reflexogenous zones passes through a continuous and transitional development from a time when a rather vigorous stimulation of any "spot" of the body within a large area serves to elicit variable, diffuse, uncoordinated patterns of behavior to a later time when a weak stimulus becomes adequate, within a much more circumscribed area for precise, well-coordinated, uniform and less variable patterns of behavior. The direction of such development is cephalocaudal.
5. The "primitive" reactions of breathing, righting, locomotion, and feeding are the products of a long and continuously progressive course of prenatal development.

6. Behavior development appears first in the gross musculature, and in the fine musculature later.

7. Behavior develops in each of the limbs from a proximal to a distal point, that is, the entire limb is first involved in the response and then gradually the more distal joints become, as it were, independent of the total movement.*

PRENATAL HUMAN DEVELOPMENT

Investigations into the field of prenatal human behavior are beset with numerous problems which were controlled or partially overcome in reported studies of infrahuman mammalian fetuses. Even when human fetuses become available for observation, it is difficult to assess the age of the fetus and this is very important both for comparative purposes and for formulating longitudinal concepts.

The starting point for the development of the new individual is taken to be the moment of fusion of the nuclei of the sperm and the ovum. However, on the basis of present knowledge, this moment cannot be accurately determined so that numerous methods have been used to calculate fetal age; namely:

1. Menstruation age where the age of the fetus is calculated from the first day of the last period of menstruation prior to the onset of pregnancy (Mall, 1918).

2. The mean menstruation age is similar to menstrual age but is based upon the average calculated from a large number of cases (Mall, 1918).

3. The conception age is calculated from the last day of the last menstrual period prior to the onset of pregnancy (Minot, 1892).

4. Copulation, or insemination, age is based upon trustworthy cases of known copulation time and upon calculation. It has been found to be approximately 10 days shorter than the mean menstrual age (Mall, 1918).

5. Ovulation age is calculated from the time of ovulation. However, since it is difficult, at present, to determine the time of

---

* (From J. D. Coronios, "Development of Behavior in the Fetal Cat," *Genet. Psychol. Monog.*, 14:283-386, 1933. By permission of the publisher, The Journal Press.)

ovulation, and the time of actual fertilization is further complicated by not knowing how long spermatozoa may survive after
entering the female genital tract, this method is not commonly
used (Hartman, 1936).

6. The fertilization, or true, age must be calculated from menstruation age, mean menstruation age, or copulation age (Mall,
1918). In general, present evidence seems to indicate that
fertilization occurs within less than 48 hours after copulation
(Carmichael, 1954).

Efforts have also been made to compile tables from which the
ages of human fetuses can be estimated from known physical measurements. However, even if organisms of truly known ages are
plentifully available, each age norm would still have to be stated
in terms of some statistical average because of the many factors, such
as genetic stock, specific pathology, and nourishment, which influence fetal size. Linear measurements of fetal specimens have been
made on the basis of crown-rump length and crown-heel length.
The former seems to be more commonly used for embryological
studies (Carmichael, 1954) while crown-heel length was used by
Minkowski (1928) in his extensive studies of human fetuses. Streeter
(1920) prepared growth curves of the human fetus based on the
relationships of weight, sitting height, foot length, head size, and
menstrual age while Hooker (1944) has suggested that weight and
length seem to provide a more useful index of behavior development than does age. In short, it would appear that the word "approximate" should appear before all statements of human fetal age
on the basis of our currently inaccurate methods of actual age
determination.

OBSERVATIONS in utero

Observations of human fetal behavior fall into two basic categories; namely, those that can be made through the body wall of
the mother and can be felt by the mother and those observations
made on fetuses which have been operatively removed for medical
reasons. The mother may sometimes perceive movements, commonly
referred to as "quickening of the fetus," as early as the seventeenth

week (Feldman, 1920). As pregnancy progresses, these movements tend to increase and to fall into three general types of fetal activity. These are quick kicks, thrusts, and jerks of the extremities; slow squirming, pushing, stretching, and turning movements; and hiccups or rhythmic series of quick convulsive movements. Figure 7 shows the results of a study by Newbery (1941) of the amount of fetal activity from the sixth to the tenth lunar month, with the greatest increases of movement occurring in the early part of this period. It is highly likely that the general reduction in activity at

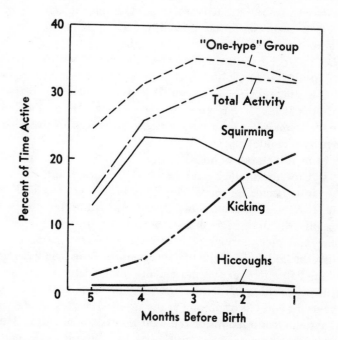

Figure 7.   Types of fetal activity. (From H. Newbery, "Studies in Fetal Behavior. IV. The Measurement of Three Types of Fetal Activity." **J. Comp. Psychol.**, 32:521-530, 1941. By permission of the publisher, The Williams and Wilkins Co.)

the end of the prenatal period is caused by the increased restriction of the growing fetus within the limiting confines of the womb and the relatively reduced oxygen and food supply.

The activity of the mother during pregnancy would also seem to influence the activity of the fetus, according to a longitudinal study conducted at the Fels Research Institute. In this instance, fetal activity was recorded, by the mothers, under different conditions of maternal activity which included eating, exercise, smoking, reading in a quiet room, and quiet interrupted by sudden noise. It was found that fatigue and emotional stress in the mother stimulated fetal activity, as did an increase in the basal metabolism rate of the mother. If such conditions prevailed over a period of time, the resultant increases in fetal activity might result in reduced birth weight and in an irritable, hypersensitive infant with gastro-intestinal dysfunction. Smoking was also found to increase the heart rate, with this effect being more marked with advancing pregnancy (Landreth, 1958). It has previously been noted that smoking by pregnant women has been associated with reduced birth weight in the newborn child.

Additional methods of observation of the fetus through the intact body wall of the mother have involved palpation and the use of various instruments for magnifying or recording various fetal movements. The most commonly used instrument is the stethoscope but, by means of suitable amplification and recording, electrocardiographic and electromyographic recordings have also been made through the body wall of the mother when the fetus is in a favorable position. Palpations of the movements of the fetus reveal similar movements to those felt by the mother. The heart beat of the fetus can be heard and felt beginning at the eighteenth week of pregnancy and rhythmic contractions of the fetal thorax, often called Ahlfeld breathing movements, have also been felt through the mother's body wall.

Conditioning of the fetus *in utero* during the last two months of pregnancy seems to have met with some success although the permanency of establishment of such conditioning is highly questionable. Spelt (1948), using a loud noise as the unconditioned stimulus which he paired with vibrotactile stimulation over the abdominal wall, reports the establishment of conditioned responses in the fetus after 15 to 20 paired stimulations. However, similar conditioning experiments in neonates reveal that conditioning is very difficult to establish and extremely unstable during this period (Pratt, 1954). The latter observations lead one to question whether the rapidity of conditioning in the fetus *in utero* is actually fetal conditioning or whether it is just a fetal manifestation induced by hormonal responses elicited by maternal conditioning.

OBSERVATIONS OF OPERATIVELY REMOVED HUMAN FETUSES

Studies of operatively removed human fetuses often give results based upon the length of the fetus rather than age. Hooker (1944) suggests that length and weight seem to provide a better index of behavior development than age. However, the temporal connotations of age are more indicative of the progressive development of behavior, so approximate age will be used in the presentation of the following observations of prenatal human behavior development.

A cautious assessment of these observations seems to be in order in view of the fact that the administration to the mother of anesthetics which permeate the placenta will influence the behavior of the fetus. Hooker (1944) found that novocain does not appear to affect the fetal movements and some of the fetuses studied by this investigator were operatively removed using only this type of anesthetic. Of particular interest is the report, by Fitzgerald and Windle (1942), of observations of three human fetuses, of approximately 8 weeks postinsemination age, which were not narcotized or anesthetized and continued to receive oxygenated blood from the intact placenta for a short period of time. They found, under these conditions, that excitability was high with quick trunk, arm, and leg movements being called out by pressing or tapping on the amniotic sac. These reactions occurred individually and in various combinations and did not involve a total reaction of the organism unless the stimulus was very strong. On the basis of these findings, these investigators concluded that an undamaged, unanesthetized or unnarcotized fetus with intact blood supply has, by the end of eight weeks, developed to the extent that its neuromuscular apparatus is capable of active functioning.

Further observations of the same fetuses after severance of the umbilical cord led to the conclusion that some receptors and synapses are more easily made nonfunctional by anoxia than others. These observations revealed that arm and leg responses have been abolished in asphyxiating specimens at a time when stimulation applied to the skin of the face still elicited trunk flexion. During this same stage of asphyxiation, it was found that strong stimulation elicited mass movements involving the trunk, arms, and legs. These findings would seem to suggest that such early mass movement in operatively removed fetuses may be a function of the decrease of oxygen in the blood and concomitant stimulation of the hypersensitive fetus.

EARLY BEHAVIORAL DEVELOPMENT

The first two weeks of prenatal viability are usually referred to as the germinal period. From the third to sixth week, called the embryonic period, the medullary groove begins to form and, within a short period of time, the primitive heart cells are laid down to begin their life-long beat in the segment which is later to become the ventricular region (Williams, 1931). This intrinsic rhythm of the heart is determined by the metabolic process of these smooth muscle cells and not by neural innervation (Goss, 1940). During this period of rapid differentiation, the cerebral and optic vesicles become recognizable and the limb buds first appear. Muscular development also proceeds rapidly at this time but at uneven rates. The smooth musculature, which is the first to develop, is clearly formed in an embryo of 1 mm. in length while the striated musculature cannot be detected in fetuses less than 2.5 mm. long.

By the sixth or seventh week of life, arms, legs, and all essential organs have been formed. From this time until birth the developing organism is called a fetus. There is considerable evidence to suggest that the onset of reaction behavior in the human fetus occurs at approximately 8 weeks of age.

Tactile stimulation in the area of the mouth of fetuses 8 to 8½ weeks of age has induced responses which spread from the very localized area of the upper lip and skin around the nostrils to the whole upper lip, chin, and part of the neck (Hooker, 1944). Contraction of the long muscles of the neck may extend downward and activate body and limb girdle muscles of the upper extremities (Hooker, 1939). Quite possibly this excitation is dependent upon the deformation of the growing tips of sensory fibers (Hogg, 1941), although receptors in the underlying tissue (Carmichael, 1954) may be activated also.

Faradic, or electrical, stimulation has also been found effective in eliciting responses (Hooker, 1939). Muscular contractions including irradiation of responses to other muscles (Minkowski, 1922) can be observed in fetuses of 8 weeks of age when stimulated in this way, but no spontaneous movements have been observed at or before this time (Hooker, 1939). These observations seem to indicate that responses to stimuli at this age are either myogenic or organized neurally at the spinal level only. Previously cited studies of infrahuman mammals indicate that musculature responds to direct stimulation before the onset of true neuromuscular action.

BEHAVIOR IN FETUSES 9 TO 12 WEEKS OF AGE

Variations in the rate of behavioral development are seen to exist at the earliest stages of fetal movement. Movements of 9 to 10 week old fetuses have been described as being slow, arrhythmical, asymmetrical and uncoordinated (Minkowski, 1921) although some reports of energetic responses by even younger fetuses have been made (Woyciechowski, 1928; Bolaffio and Artom, 1924).

Spontaneous movements have been reported in fetuses of approximately 9 weeks of age (Woyciechowski, 1928; Hooker, 1939) although the origin of such movement is not fully understood. It is generally believed that even during the third month the cerebral cortex has not yet assumed any functions in relation to general bodily activity. Bolaffio and Artom (1924) did report an instance in which decerebration of an 8½ week fetus resulted in greater vividness of response, apparently indicating even at this stage some inhibition by the cortex on lower reflexes. These same investigators found that mechanical stimulation of the medulla led to respiratory movements and to a primitive form of sucking. Some immature connections between the brain and the periphery have evidently been established at this time.

The general observation is made by Hooker (1944) that during the period from 9½ to 12 weeks in fetal development a "total pattern" or response to stimuli is dominant. He found, for example, that at 11 weeks of age stimulation of the mouth area brought a response from the entire upper extremity and even the sole of the foot. Minkowski's anatomical studies (1928) show that the spinal cord and nerve trunks have no medullary sheaths before the 12th week and this may provide a partial explanation of the spread of response.

Reflex action becomes increasingly evident in the developing organism, however. Stretching of limb muscles is effective in stimulating proprioceptive organs and eliciting a response at 9½ weeks. At 11 weeks, palmar stimulation results in a quick but incomplete finger closure, apparently marking the onset of the grasping reflex. At this same period, the plantar reflex and patterned eye movements can be identified (Hooker, 1944). It was previously noted (Windle and Fitzgerald, 1937) that the spinal reflex arcs are developed by the 8th week. Specific functions can be elicited increasingly thereafter.

BEHAVIOR IN FETUSES 13 TO 16 WEEKS OF AGE

By 13 weeks, almost every joint in the body that is ever to move has gained motility (Hooker, 1944) and this fact, of course, makes it possible to observe the results of stimulation over the entire range of joint action. Strong stimulation will result in what is sometimes called a "generalized matrix of behavior" while weak stimulation of certain receptor areas leads to very specific responses. Carmichael (1951) points to the importance of vestibular and proprioceptive stimuli in establishing the postural tone of the body which in turn will affect the type of response that is elicited by any particular stimuli at any particular time. He notes that when the head is turned to one side the response may not be the same as when the head is turned to the other side. Furthermore, stimulation of the sole of the foot at this age may result in either flexion or extension of the toes depending upon the posture of the toes at the time of stimulation (Sherman and Sherman, 1925).

On the basis of our knowledge of the summation of impulses required for response at different neural levels, it is conceivable the neural mechanisms may be available at this time to allow for differentiation in response according to the strength of the stimulus and its locus. Minkowski (1922) reports that touching the tongue or lower lip of a fetus approximately 13 weeks old with a blunt probe resulted in the closure of the mouth. He also observed prominent reflexes of the trunk and extremities in this fetus but found that these were discontinued at once following transection of the spinal cord in the dorsal region. These results seem to prove that for this fetus at this age conduction of activation was through innervation of the spinal cord. Minkowski made the further observation that, following transection of the spinal cord, the short reflexes remained unchanged. These, however, were also abolished following total extirpation of the cord. During the course of this experiment, it was noted that destruction of the cervical cord abolished reflexes of the arms while destruction of the lumbar and sacral cord resulted in the abolition of reflexes in the legs. It would appear, then, that after the 13th week the reflex response in the human infant can, in general, no longer be considered as being on the simple two-neuron arc level but is now subject to an increasing number of modifying influences.

The development of some of the reflex responses requiring more complex neural innervation seems to be a major aspect of behavioral development during this period. Spontaneous movements have been observed at 14 weeks of age which include most body parts as well as activity of the "organism as a whole" with movements elicited by tactual stimulation being characterized as "graceful" and "delicate." Except for the true grasping reflex, respiration, vocalization, and a few others, the fetus at this age shows most of the specific patterns of response that can be found in the neonate (Hooker, 1944). Although contralateral responses have been observed in a limited way during the ninth week (Fitzgerald and Windle, 1942), it is not until approximately 13 weeks of age that stimulation of receptor fields on one side of the body regularly leads to the response of a limb on the

other side of the body (Hooker, 1944). Definite indications of reciprocal innervation during movement of a limb were noted in a fetus
of about 16 weeks by Minkowski (1924) who also reports the establishment of diagonal reflexes at this time. Here, stimulation of one
foot of the fetus led to movement of the arm on the opposite side
and Minkowski considered these observations of diagonal reflexes as
being significant in comparing the ontogenetic development of the
human fetus with the trotting reflex noted by observers of infrahuman fetal development.

BEHAVIOR DEVELOPMENT FROM 17 WEEKS
TO NORMAL BIRTH

In general, the period from 17 weeks until normal birth is marked
by the increasing dominance of the central nervous system in the
behavior responses of the human fetus. Direct mechanical stimulation of the motor roots of the spinal nerve in a fetus of approximately 17 weeks indicated that intersegmental spinal conduction
had become well established. This particular fetus responded to
mechanical stimulation of the cranial nerves at the level of the
medulla by opening and closing of the mouth, presumably the result of direct stimulation of the facial nerve. Stimulation of the
medulla itself resulted in changes in the Ahlfeld breathing movements but direct stimulation of the cortex did not elicit any responses (Minkowski, 1922). Mechanical stimulation of the Rolandic
zone of the brain of another fetus of similar age did not call forth
any reaction but removal of the cerebral hemispheres did result in
more vivid responses to local stimuli than had been elicited previously. In this fetus, respiratory movements in response to stimulation of the medulla were so violent that they led to elevation of the
shoulder and the adduction of the arms (Bolaffio and Artom, 1924).
It would appear, then, that the respiratory mechanisms seated in the
medulla have achieved effective neural connections after approximately 17 weeks and that intersegmental spinal conduction of other
reflexes is also well established at this level.

Rhythmic chest movements were first reported in 1890 by Ahlfeld,
who noted that the responses varied from 38 to 76 per minute. This
timing and the rhythmicity of the movements tends to indicate

that the breathing mechanism is essentially in working order long before it is needed (Carmichael, 1954). These respiratory movements of the fetus do not normally lead to aspiration of the amniotic fluid (Windle, 1941) and some investigators have suggested that the rhythmic movements act as a sort of auxilliary pump to help the heart in its function (Carmichael, 1954). It is also considered likely that a decrease in the oxygen content of the fetal blood may be one of the causes of these movements. Richards et al. (1938) observed intact fetuses through the maternal wall during the last 20 weeks of pregnancy and, following continuous observations for 5 to 6 hours, noted a correlation of .60 between chest movements and the metabolic rate of the mother. Although at 22 weeks, some prematurely delivered fetuses are capable of briefly sustaining respiration when stimulated by air, it is not until the sixth to seventh month that the respiratory mechanism ordinarily becomes sufficiently established to permanently maintain respiration.

Response to electrical stimulation of the brain at the level of the pons is not reported until approximately 5 months fetal age when such stimulation resulted in synchronous responses from the muscles innervated by the facial nerve. Here, stimulation of the medulla also resulted in energetic respiratory movements while stimulation of the cervical cord elicited energetic elevation of the shoulders together with flexion of the arms. Stimulation of the lumbar cord led to movements of the legs (Bolaffio and Artom, 1924). In fetuses of approximately 6 months of age, stimulation of the lower brain centers resulted in increased rate of respiratory movements and in shoulder, arm, and finger movements. However, stimulation of the cerebral cortex itself still produced negative results, although removal of the cortex resulted in the usual response of heightened reaction to sensory stimulation (Bolaffio and Artom, 1924). These findings, together with the known susceptibility of neural tissue to oxygen deficiency, suggest that the increases in vividness of responses to stimulation by fetuses just before death are attributable to changes in the higher brain centers.

The tracing of behavioral responses to stimulation of the sole of the foot from the time of onset of reaction to the elicitation of the adult plantar reflex is illustrative of the fact that the same stimuli applied to the same area may call out differing, yet quite specific, responses as the various connecting levels of the nervous system mature. Minkowski (1926) believes that the first response to stimulation of the sole of the foot is probably myogenic, produced by direct stimulation of the muscle through the thin skin, and thus does not involve any neural elements. The dorsal flexion of the toes which occurs during the third and fourth months in response to stimulation is believed to involve connections in the spinal cord. With the continuing maturation of the central nervous system and the development of effective connections to the midbrain during the midfetal period, the pattern of response changes to one of big toe extension with the other toes being flexed. Subsequent development of still higher nerve centers in later fetal life results in variable responses, one of which may be spreading of the toes. The typical Babinski reflex (big toe extension and flexion of the other toes) disappears shortly after birth with the development of cortical dominance. The adult plantar reflex (contraction of all toes) is associated with the development of cortical dominance and any reversion to, or retention of, the Babinski reflex is considered to be indicative of a lesion of the pyramidal tracts of the brain and the spinal cord (Pratt, 1954).

The trend toward increased localization of response continues as the fetus becomes older. One must, however, inject reservations into such a general statement based upon the nature and the strength of the stimuli. For example, superficial stimulation elicited localized muscular contractions in the limbs and in other specialized muscle groups in a fetus of approximately 19 weeks while strong deep stimulation of a single segment of one limb resulted in flexion of the whole contralateral limb (Bolaffio and Artom, 1924). Specificity of response tends to be more marked in the head region than in the leg region in fetuses of approximately 22 weeks (Bolaffio and Artom, 1924), with very specific activation of the muscles of the eyelid occurring in response to a single electrical stimulus (Minkowski, 1922). Vivid reaction has been obtained from all the muscles of the limbs when they are excited one at a time by percussion in a fetus of approximately 24 weeks (Bolaffio and Artom, 1924).

During the sixth month, fetuses have exhibited responses which may be classified as the first tendon reflexes rather than responses to cutaneous or muscle stimulation. Bolaffio and Artom (1924) base their recognition of the onset of true tendon reflexes at this time upon the facts that the specific responses elicited by stimuli were not observed previously and that the responses were similar to those elicited as true tendon reflexes in early infancy. Furthermore, once these responses were capable of being elicited, they continued to increase in strength during the remainder of the fetal period. During the next two months of pregnancy, muscular reflexes tend to decrease in their ascendancy over the tendon reflexes until, by the end of the ninth month, the tendon reflexes are so well established that they prevail over special muscle reflexes. With the exception of some tendon reflexes of the upper limbs which are difficult to elicit because of the small size of the limb, all tendon reflexes are found to be present during this period of life. Some of the earlier developing tendon reflexes are the biceps, triceps, and Achilles tendon reflexes and the knee jerk.

The increase in the elaboration of the types of responses together with more precise differentiation of the muscular responses during this period is indicative of the maturation of the neural mechanisms in terms of elaboration of neural connections and maturation of the various neural components. By the seventh month, certain responses have been characterized as involving synergic muscle groups (Bolaffio and Artom, 1924). Although the activity of the newborn has been classified as "mass activity" (Irwin and Weiss, 1930), the movement during such activity is not similar to the diffuse type of response noted by investigators of the early fetal period. Certainly by the end of the seventh month myelinization of all the fundamental activities pathways is almost complete and the myelinization of the other motor pathways is in progress (Minkowski, 1928). On the basis of these findings, it seems unlikely that one can still attribute "mass activity" to the spread of responses because of lack of medullary sheaths as may be the case prior to the fourth fetal month.

Faint sounds indicative of the onset of vocal function are reported in a fetus of approximately 22 weeks (Minkowski, 1922) while weak crying sounds were made by another fetus of about 25 weeks of age (Bolaffio and Artom, 1924). Corneal reflexes have been observed in the seventh month with direct stimulation of the cornea eliciting increasingly stronger responses as the fetus grows older (Minkowski,

1922). During the last month of pregnancy iris reflexes have been noted but the response of the iris is very slow and a very strong light is required before the reaction is elicited (Minkowski, 1928). Variations in the grasping reflex are reported by Bolaffio and Artom (1924), who noted that very light stimulation of the hand results in variable and inconstant responses while strong stimulation, which may because of its strength involve the muscles or underlying tissues, uniformly elicits grasping. On the basis of such observations, these investigators concluded that the grasping reflex should not be considered as a purely cutaneous reflex in prenatal life.

It would appear, then, that all processes vital for the survival of the fetus are firmly established before the last two months of pregnancy. The heart beat, with its role in the circulatory system, and the respiratory mechanisms have been discussed. Peristaltic movements of the digestive tract, swallowing of amniotic fluid, and excretion of urine have also been developing gradually since the first half of the pregnancy period. The fetus, therefore, has achieved, by the seventh month of pregnancy, the age of viability although some of the reflexes of later fetal life may not be functional as yet. A summary of the responses of a full-term newborn infant includes the following: eyelid, pupillary, ocular, tear secretion, facial and mouth, throat, neck, head, arm, trunk, foot, and leg, and the coordinate position of many of the parts of the body (Dennis, 1934). Some of these responses will be discussed in greater detail in the chapter on the neonate. Suffice it to say here that the vast changes that have occurred from the original fertilized ovum to the newborn child during the short period of 280 days still stagger the human imagination—one of the ultimate products of this development.

Briefly, and in general, prenatal behavioral development in the human fetus may be classified as:

1. Rapid, progressive, and continuous, with variations in rate occurring between individuals.
2. Very generally, behavior development progresses from weak, diffuse, massive, relatively unorganized responses to a condition where many reactions are stronger, more specific in nature, and better organized.
3. Prenatal development of behavior appears to progress along a cephalocaudal course as does also the development of reflex-

ogenous zones. It appears that myogenic responses precede true sensory responses and that proprioceptive mechanisms seem to be functional before the onset of function in the cutaneous system.

4. Development of essential life functions involves a long, continuous process and is completed well in advance of the time when they will be required by the newborn infant to sustain independent existence.

5. Behavior development appears first in the gross musculature and later in the fine musculature.

6. Behavior tends to develop in the limbs in a proximal to distal direction. These latter two statements must be considered broad generalizations in that it is exceedingly difficult to apply stimulation to minute, specific areas of very young fetuses because of their small size.

The generalization that ontogeny recapitulates phylogeny has been noted at various times in the previous presentation. This would appear to hold for histological and morphological development but is questionable if an attempt is made to apply it to the development of locomotion in the human being. While there is a general relationship in the sequence of development of behavioral capacities from fish to man and investigations have shown that the first responses in fish, amphibians, and the lower mammals involve a lateral bending of the trunk, no observations have, as yet, been made where the first trunk movements in the human fetus are unaccompanied by arm movements. Moreover, the locomotor mechanisms of fish and amphibians require a high degree of trunk muscle integration that does not appear to be similar to the neuromotor requirements for bipedal locomotion in man. Furthermore, the great variation in the creeping behavior of infants and the lack of evidence of rhythm in the movements of the limbs of the human fetus lends little support to the generalization of ontogeny recapitulating phylogeny in the development of human locomotion.

CHAPTER V

THE NEONATE

The process of birth, which, under normal conditions, involves the contraction of the uterus so that the fetal membranes are ruptured and the developing child is expelled through the birth canal, severs the parasitic connections of the child with the mother and necessitates the autonomous functioning of the child's vegetative systems if it is to survive. As previously pointed out all the systems required for the sustenance of life are operative about two months prior to normal birth. However, the change from a liquid environment to a gaseous one means that there has been no opportunity for the respiratory system to function normally prior to the crucial time at birth when it must function or the child will be asphyxiated. Furthermore, the agent, or agents, which initiate the act of breathing become vitally important at this time.

Studies of conditions surrounding the onset of breathing indicate that the increase in metabolites and carbon dioxide together with a decrease in the oxygen content of the blood are important factors in causing the first gasps following severance of the umbilical cord

(Corey, 1931). Other investigations show that external stimuli such as the drying of the skin and its cooling are also important factors in initiating the first breath (Barcroft and Karvonen, 1948). In this connection, a slap is sometimes effective if a baby does not start breathing upon delivery (Huggett, 1930). Barcroft et al. (1940) contend that movements of the respiratory type seem to arise from the release of an inhibitory center in the forebrain.

The birth experience itself has been considered by some psycho-analysts to be traumatic but no evidence is available to support this claim except in the case of birth injury and here it is probably the injury itself that must be considered responsible rather than the birth as such. In an attempt to assess the effects of the birth experi-ence, Ruja (1948) studied the relationship between the length of labor and crying in newborn infants. Although a positive relation-ship was found, the results may be questioned, as crying was meas-ured on different infants at different intervals from 1 to 8 days after birth. Pratt et al. (1930), in a continuous study of crying in newborn infants, found that crying normally increases during the first 10 days regardless of the length of labor. This increase might be expected in the light of findings, based on electroencephalograms, that the administration of sodium seconal during labor resulted in reduced cortical activity in the infant even after all clinical signs of drowsi-ness had disappeared (Hughes et al., 1948). Such reduced cortical activity may well be reflected in lowered reactions, including crying, during the first days after birth. It should be noted, however, that neonatal behavior is often considered subcortical since the cortex is relatively undeveloped at birth.

On the positive side, Ashley Montagu (1962) contends that labor provides a stimulant for the autonomic systems, particularly the respiratory and urogenital. His observations of children and adults who were delivered by Ceasarean section has led him to the con-clusion that these individuals are more likely to suffer respiratory and urogenital dysfunction.

Although there are some unanswered questions concerning the effects of the birth experience itself, there is certainly no doubt that the rapid transition from a protected, parasitic existence to autono-mous survival in the external world is a physiological strain on the neonate. The following briefly summarizes the main areas of transition that must be achieved by the child from prenatal to postnatal life.

*Variables of Prenatal and Postnatal Life**

	Prenatal	Postnatal
Physical environment	Fluid (amniotic).	Gaseous (air).
External temperature	Approximately constant.	Fluctuates with external conditions.
Oxygen supply	Hemotrophic; diffusion through the placenta.	From lung surface to blood stream.
Nutrition	Hemotrophic; dependent on nutrients in mother's blood.	Based on available food and functioning of digestive tract. Indigestible wastes must be eliminated.
Elimination of products of metabolism	Into maternal blood stream.	Elimination by lungs, skin, and kidneys.
Sensory stimulation	At minimum except for kinesthetic and vibratory.	All sense modalities stimulated by a variety of stimuli.

* From Catherine Landreth, *The Psychology of Early Childhood*. New York: Alfred A. Knopf, 1958. By permission of the author.

The immense degree of adjustment that occurs in the vegetative functions with birth is reflected in many cases by a loss of weight during the first 3 days which may not be recovered until the end of the tenth day. Another indication of the physiological strain imposed upon the infant at birth is the mortality rate, which is higher during the first 10 days than at any subsequent period. Indeed, the neonatal period must be considered as a period of adjustment and perfection of the newly activated physiological and sensory functions.

A few investigators in the field of infant development have considered the neonatal period as extending to approximately the end of the first week after birth; others consider it to include the first 2 postnatal weeks; still others place its duration as the first month with the extreme being the first 3 months. Most current usage in the field of infant behavior tends to consider the neonatal period as encompassing the first postnatal month as this time period would seem to be sufficient for the adjustment and perfection of the newly activated functions and for recovery from injuries such as asphyxia, obstetrical paralysis, umbilical infections, and hemorrhages incurred during birth (Pratt, 1954).

AUTONOMIC SYSTEMS

Comprehensive investigations of heart beat and pulse rate of the neonate have reported great variation under different conditions. During sleep the average pulse rate was found to be 123.5 per minute with the rate being some 94.7 beats higher during crying (Halverson, 1941). Observations through the maternal wall during the last month before birth indicate that vibratory stimuli applied to the abdomen of the mother increased the average heart rate by approximately 14.3 beats per minute. Furthermore, similar observations revealed that smoking by the mother increased the fetal heart beat approximately 5 beats per minute some 8 to 12 minutes after smoking was started (Sontag and Wallace, 1936). Therefore, stimuli of different modalities appear to produce considerable variation in pulse rate both in the fetus and in the neonate.

Although it is sometimes assumed that the birth cry is the first respiratory response of the neonate, observations based upon high speed motion pictures indicate that gasping is the first respiratory response after birth (Schmidt, 1950; Peiper, 1951). Schmidt (1950) found that gasping lasted from 13 to 45 seconds in normal full-term infants but increased in duration to 6½ minutes in premature 8-month infants and up to 12 minutes in difficult births. Following the initial respiratory gasp, the breathing rate is, as is the heart rate, subject to a great deal of variation depending upon internal and external stimuli. There is also a marked variation from one infant to the other with the average rate during sleep prior to awakening being 32.3 breaths per minute and rising to a maximal average of 133.3 respirations per minute during crying (Halverson, 1941).

Other responses intimately associated with respiration such as yawning, coughing, and sneezing are reported to occur shortly after birth while the birth cry itself is considered to be a concomitant of the initiation of pulmonary respiration. There is a relationship between the centers governing the respiratory, sucking, and swallowing reflexes during the sucking period of the infant such that the child is able to suck, swallow, and breathe at the same time—a facility which he will later lose as it is not possessed by adults. It is believed that the swallowing center influences the sucking center which, in turn, influences the rhythm of the breathing center (Peiper, 1939). Both Peiper (1939) and Halverson (1944) have found that swallowing occurs during the phases between breathing with the latter investigator also reporting that sucking occurs simultaneously with breathing except during strong sucking when the sucks tend to come after inspiration. Good coordination of these centers appears even in premature infants.

The transition from maternally supplied nutrient materials to independent assimilation of nutrients by means of the alimentary tract in the neonate may be one cause of an initial loss of weight. Other possible causes may be imperfect assimilation, or the possibility that colostrum does not meet the energy requirements of the newborn infant. In some cases the scantiness of the maternal milk production may be responsible. Under optimum conditions, no loss of weight may occur although there are wide individual differences in infant adjustment.

The neonate exhibits mouth orientation, or seeking, responses which are elicited by tactual stimulation of the lip and adjacent face areas and result in the bringing of the opened mouth to the nipple. When contact is properly established, sucking begins and the ingestion of food follows. Salivation is firmly established in the neonate and is initiated by sucking. As previously mentioned, sucking, breathing, and swallowing are coordinated so that the passage of food to the stomach presents no problem to the suckling. Arrival of the food in the stomach stimulates gastric secretion and when the stomach becomes filled the child ceases nursing. After the infant has ceased nursing and broken contact with the nipple, there is frequently some regurgitation of food which, in turn, is often followed by hiccuping.

The stomach of the neonate has been found to empty in 4 to 5 hours at the most; the intestines in 7 or 8 hours; and the large intestine within 2 to 14 hours. Carlson and Ginsburg (1915) have demonstrated, by using a balloon on the stomach of infants prior to nursing, that "hunger" contractions, similar to those found in adults, occur in the neonate. However, during the first 2 weeks, "hunger" contractions in normal full-term infants begin in the stomach about 2 hours and 50 minutes after the previous nursing period. During the period from the 2nd to 8th week, the time duration increases until contractions start at about 3 hours and 40 minutes after nursing. These observations would indicate that the "hunger" contractions arise before the stomach has been emptied and cannot, therefore, be ascribed to an empty stomach.

These muscular contractions of the stomach are more vigorous in the neonate than in the adult with observations revealing a concomitant increase in reflex excitability that was synchronous with the periods of stomach contractions. Although, in the adult, the contractions may be inhibited by introducing taste substances in the mouth, in the neonate they are only temporarily inhibited by the administration of small quantities of water or milk (Taylor, 1917). After observing 73 infants, Irwin (1932) found that general motility correlated .97 with the elapsed time between feeding periods. Bodily oscillations measured on a stabilometer during the first 15 minutes after feeding averaged 17.0 per minute while during the last 15 minutes period prior to nursing the oscillations soared to approximately 45 per minute.

The sequence of activities in the alimentary canal is completed by egestion or defecation. The first half hour after feeding is the period during which defecation occurs most frequently with the modal number of defecations being approximately 5 in 24 hours (Halverson, 1940). Most defecations occur during wakefulness with the infant being active before and during the act and quiescent following the act (Pratt, 1954). The activity associated with defecation is greater than the activity prior to micturition which occurs approximately 18 times during a 24 hour period. As with defecation, the greatest number of micturitions occur within the first hour after feeding and during periods of wakefulness with completion of the act resulting in quiescence (Halverson, 1940). On the basis of his own and other investigators' observations, Pratt (1954) believes it is possible that a great deal of the young infant's general motility is in some way dependent upon the alimentary processes.

SLEEP

Numerous investigators have studied the sleep of newborn infants using different criteria for defining sleep. The oldest and most widely used has been the closure of the eyes although the criterion of decreased irritability and activity is currently being accepted as a more valid indicator. The neonate sleeps 20 hours out of 24 with the duration of each sleep period being no more than 3 hours and usually less (Pratt et al., 1930). Contrary to usual belief, more infants are awake during the first 15 minutes after feeding than during the last 15 minutes prior to the next nursing period with most infants being asleep during the middle 15 minutes between nursing periods (Irwin, 1932). The depth of sleep is variable from one infant to another and it varies according to the condition and the activities of the infant prior to falling asleep. As the child grows older, the total hours of sleep decrease but the length of each sleep period increases so that longer periods of wakefulness gradually supplant periods of sleep. In contrast with the amount of stimulation required to awaken the neonate, it has been found that weaker electrical stimuli will awaken the child as it grows older (Pratt, 1954). In this regard, it should be pointed out that most investigations of the responses of the neonate are carried out with quiescent infants so that the effects of the experimental stimuli will not be masked by other activity and may, on the basis of the simple criterion of sleep being reduced motility, be regarded as involving sleeping infants.

BODILY POSTURES

Rather well-defined resting and sleeping postures have been observed in the neonate. The arms and legs tend to be flexed and the fists clenched with even the most marked extension, such as the upper arms at right angles to the body and the forearms parallel to the head, still exhibiting some flexion. Gesell and Thompson (1938) reported that all of the infants examined in their normative survey spontaneously maintained the head predominantly rotated to one side at 4 weeks of age. All the infants also held their arms in the tonic neck reflex attitude which involves extension of the arm on the side to which the head is turned together with flexion of the opposite arm. On the basis of these observations, these investigators concluded that the tonic neck reflex is a normal feature of neonatal infancy.

The positionings of the neonate are, in a sense, also conditioned by the previous confinement within the fetal membranes, where full extension of the limbs was impossible, and by the body proportions and muscular strength of the newborn infant. At birth, the average infant is approximately 20 inches long from the crown of the head to the heel and weighs approximately 7½ pounds. The head, with its large cranium and relatively small face, makes up one-fourth of the body length and is too heavy to be supported easily in a vertical position when the infant is placed on its back. The body, with the chest circumference approximately the same as the diameter of the head, takes up one-half of the remaining total length so that the arms and legs are relatively short in comparison with adult body proportions. The major portion of the mass of the newborn infant, is therefore, composed of the head and body so that any action of the weak limbs is ineffective with respect to motility of the body as a whole.

SENSORY SYSTEMS

The neonatal period marks the first time certain sensory-motor structures are activated by adequate stimuli with this stimulation in turn helping to bring about further maturation of the nervous system. The reactivity of the sensory-motor structures reveals the effects of fetal maturation but does not, in itself, induce profound developmental events or provide a basis for more than the mere beginnings of learning. The responsiveness of the neonate to internal stimuli has already been discussed in relation to the functioning of the alimentary tract. It may be recalled that the internal stimuli tend to have a rhythmic incidence and to occur over periods of fairly long duration. It is believed the transition from fetal to postnatal existence may involve a greater stepping up of internal than of external stimuli. On the basis of previously cited observa-

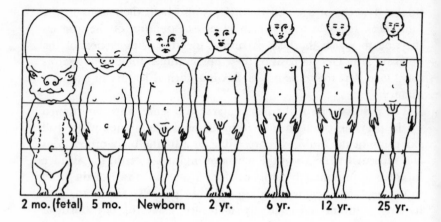

| 2 mo. (fetal) | 5 mo. | Newborn | 2 yr. | 6 yr. | 12 yr. | 25 yr. |

Figure 8.   Changes in form and proportion of the human
                body during fetal and post-natal life. (From
                C. M. Jackson, "Some Aspects of Form and
                Growth." In W. J. Robbins, S. Brody, A. G.
                Hogan, C. M. Jackson, and C. W. Green,
                Growth. New Haven: Yale University Press,
                1928. By permission of the publisher.)

tions of motility in the neonate, it would appear that stimuli associated with internal processes would account for most of the
infant's motility. Investigations of the role of external stimuli indicate that the responses vary according to the type, intensity, and
duration of the stimulus but are always set against the background
of internal stimuli and tend to add little to the total activity. Moreover, in some instances, it has been found that external stimuli will
reduce total activity.

VISION

There is little doubt that the newborn infant has some vision but
the extent of such vision is still problematic. Coordinate compensatory eye-movements have been observed as soon as 32 hours after
birth (Ling, 1942) and pupillary reflexes are present at birth. With
increased age, an increase in sensitivity of pupillary responses is

shown with less intense stimuli being required to elicit responses (Sherman et al., 1936). The most invariable type of response aroused by visual stimuli is the visuopalpebral reflex which involves the closing, tightening, or twitching of closed eyelids and is elicited by flashes of light (Pratt et al., 1930). Another response to a flash of light, the ocular-neck involving a bending backwards of the head, is dependent upon the intensity of light (Peiper, 1926). Bright, intense flashes of light have been observed to release Moro or "startle" reflexes as well as ocular-neck, pupillary, visuopalpebral, circulatory, and respiratory responses with the incidence of the Moro or "startle" reflexes being higher during the first few days of the neonatal period (Pratt et al., 1930).

Although the immediate responses to light changes of various intensities is excitatory and there is no apparent differentiation according to intensity, prolonged periods of illumination of the same intensity have been found to result in decreased activity (Weiss, 1934). Sudden reduction of visual stimuli, such as when the infant is subjected to darkness after having been exposed to an illumination of 5 foot-candles for a period of five minutes, results in an increase in activity (Irwin, 1941). However, the infant soon adapts to the dark and, once adaptation is complete, will respond with increased sensitivity to visual stimuli which would normally be inadequate to elicit responses from a light-adapted eye (Peiper, 1926).

The onset of visual pursuit movements has been placed at one (Beasley, 1933) and two weeks (McGinnis, 1930) by different observers with horizontal pursuit movements tending to appear before vertical and circular pursuit movements. There are variations in the responses from one infant to another with respect to the optimum rate of movement and the distance of the moving light from the eyes (Beasley, 1933). On the basis of duration and fixation of gaze, it is generally accepted that the neonate has color vision with the gaze tending to rest longest on blue and green, shortest on yellow, while red comes in between (Stirnimann, 1944).

HEARING

The neonate is capable of hearing as it responds to auditory stimuli in such ways as quivering of the eyelids, head movements, wrinkling of the forehead, crying, and awakening from sleep. Louder stimuli produce more bodily movements, increases in respiratory and heart action and greater frequency of eyelid closure (Stubbs, 1934) while, as with visual stimuli, auditory stimuli of long durations, such as 5 minutes, tend to decrease bodily movements significantly in comparison with periods during which no stimuli are presented (Weiss, 1934). The most frequent reaction to auditory stimuli is the acoustopalpebral reflex which is similar in nature to the visuopalpebral reflex (Froeschels and Bebbe, 1946) with the Moro or "startle" response being elicited by sudden, loud noises. The physiological condition of the neonate has a definite effect on the responses to auditory stimuli with stimuli being most easily elicited during sleep and most difficult to activate during nursing (Pratt, 1954). The smallest percentages of responses are obtained when infants are crying and the greatest number when they are awake and inactive (Stubbs, 1934).

SMELL AND TASTE

Determination of the extent of olfactory sensitivity in the neonate is hampered by methodological difficulties in assessing purely olfactory stimulation. Although vocalization, facial responses, and general bodily movement have been observed in response to ammonia and acetic acid fumes and sucking responses have been noted in response to the fumes of valerian, it is difficult to know whether these responses should be attributed to olfactory stimulation or to irritation of the mucous membrane of the nose (Pratt et al. 1930).

Taste is considered to be highly developed in the neonate but it is uncertain whether all four taste qualities are fully differentiated. Of all gustatory stimuli tests, only salt solutions impaired sucking responses or caused them to cease (Jensen, 1932) whereas sucking responses are most pronounced in response to the administration of sugar solutions and are found to increase in prominence in this category with age (Pratt et al., 1930). Furthermore, the degree of satiation also affects the response, with the moderately full infant being a better discriminator of gustatory stimuli than the hungry one.

CUTANEOUS SENSITIVITY

Thermal sensitivity seems to be well developed in the neonate. Numerous investigations of various parts of the body indicate great variability from one area to another but suggest the possibility that the legs and feet are more sensitive to thermal stimulation than the head and hand areas (Pratt, 1954). It would also appear that different areas of the body have different high and low temperature thresholds where stimuli deviating from these thresholds will elicit vigorous responses. Furthermore, a definite preference for certain temperatures is indicated by the seeking movements of one foot towards the other when the latter is being subjected to a warm stimulation while a relatively cold stimulus will result in the withdrawal of the stimulated limb (Stirnimann, 1939). General environmental temperatures have been reported as giving rise to shivering (Blanton, 1917) and a correlation of −.205 has been obtained between environmental temperatures and general activity in the infant (Pratt, 1930). A study by Irwin and Weiss (1934) of 50 clothed and unclothed infants indicated less crying by the former with the conclusion being that clothing provides some thermal insulation from atmospheric stimuli.

Sensitivity to contact or pressure stimuli is well developed in the newborn infant but it is difficult to differentiate the effects of these stimuli from the effects of pain, thermal, or other stimuli. Although there have been no systematic investigations of the differences in tactual sensitivity of all of the cutaneous surfaces of the neonate's body, the results of numerous studies tend to suggest the face, hands, and the soles of the feet as having the greatest sensitivity while the shoulders, back, breast, and abdomen have the least. In assessing cutaneous reflexes, the investigator is also faced with the problem of controlling the intensity of the stimulus so as to be sure the response elicited is purely cutaneous and does not also involve pressure sensory receptors (Pratt, 1954). Furthermore, responses to similar stimuli will change with the age of the child (Nassau, 1938). In general, the response evoked from any given body area by tactual stimuli will vary with their intensity and duration, the physiological condition of the infant, and whether the application of the stimulus involves stroking or punctiform contact. The responses elicited range from local reflexes to general body movements and include palpebral, pupillary, Moro, startle, tonic neck, withdrawal, and plantar responses.

Additional responses to tactual stimuli provide a fundamental orientation of the infant to its surroundings. Of primary importance in this regard is the mouth orientation response of the infant to contact stimulation of the cheek which was noted above in relation to sucking. Stimulation above or below the lips will result in the throwing back of the head or the dropping of the chin according to the respective area of stimulation. There are variations in the extent of these responses depending upon the locale of the area stimulated with the lips, above the lips, below the lips, and the cheek being decreasingly sensitive in the order listed. The sensitivity of the cheek area tends to decrease with age (Pratt, 1954).

Response to pain stimuli has been recorded in the neonate but the differential sensitivity of the various areas of the body has not been fully investigated. Even for those areas investigated, there is some disagreement as to the relative sensitivity of the areas. One group of investigators has found the head areas to be more sensitive than the leg areas (Sherman et al., 1936) whereas another group noted that the head areas were least sensitive, the arms more so, with the legs being most sensitive (Dockeray and Rice, 1934). The relative sensitivity of the newborn to pain in comparison with the later neonatal period is also an area in which variable observations have been recorded. In one instance, investigation of newly born infants over a period of time indicated a decrease in the average number of pin pricks required to elicit a response in both the head and the leg regions over the first few days (Sherman and Sherman, 1925) while, in another instance, no change in response was found with age during the neonatal period (Dockeray and Rice, 1934).

KINESTHETIC SENSITIVITY

Sensitivity to movement or changes in body position are exhibited in the neonate by movements of the body as a whole or by various parts of the body. Sudden loss of support, sudden elevation of the body, and sudden jarring of the surface upon which the infant is resting result in the elicitation of the Moro or "startle" response. In these instances, the response is considered to be conditioned by static-kinesthetic sensitivity whereby the spatial movement stimulates the static receptors to elicit the response. Some investigators have expressed the opinion that the generalized responses of the newborn infant may be touched off indirectly by static-kinesthetic sensitivity to the more local responses set off directly by other stimuli (Pratt, 1954).

GENERAL RESPONSES

The Moro response is a general bodily response to sudden, strong light and sound as well as static-kinesthetic sensitivity. Moro, in 1918, described this response as a clasping response which consists of the symmetrical extension of the arms followed by their bowing and return to the body with the legs undergoing the same kind of movement although their involvement may not be so great (Pratt, 1954). Subsequent investigators have deemed that the Moro response is not a true clasping or embracing response as the extended arms do not hold or clasp the experimenter's arm and that it is a variation of the "startle" response which is a purely flexion response. Both patterns of response are clearly present at 6 weeks of age but the Moro disappears after a few months, whereas the startle response persists into adult life (Landis and Hunt, 1939).

Rotation of the body in a horizontal plane has been found to result in compensatory head movements in the same direction during rotation followed by movement in the opposite direction after cessation of rotation (McGraw, 1941b). Turning of an infant's head to the side suddenly when it is lying on its back results in the adoption of the "fencing" posture of the tonic neck reflex while passive flexion of one leg of the infant when it is lying on its back will automatically result in the flexion of the other leg (Pratt, 1954). Responses during inversion, when the infant is suspended by the ankles, indicate a momentary backward bending of the head resulting from contraction in the cervical region (Irwin, 1936) and a flexion of the knees and of the hip resulting in an up-and-down motion of the body (McGraw, 1940b). Some investigators consider these responses to be related to early attempts at locomotion (Mc-Graw, 1946). General body position during inverted suspension consists of the head and body being roughly aligned in the vertical plane and the arms being maintained in their usual flexed position.

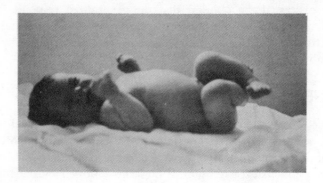

Figure 9.   Normal term infant at 4 weeks of age.

In general, the newborn infant is completely dominated by gravity, since it does not have the strength to hold its head or trunk upright or in alignment when suspended at the abdomen, buttocks, or at the side of the hip. It is also unable to maintain a sitting posture when placed in a sitting position but is able, as with inverted suspension, to momentarily lift its head when placed in a prone position on a solid surface. A newborn infant will also make alternate, or "stepping" movements when held in an erect posture with its feet resting on a surface. The latter two activities have been regarded as the first indicators of future upright, bipedal locomotion although McGraw (1946), one of the earliest investigators to assign locomotory implications to these responses, believes that genuine upright ambulation is impossible in the neonate because of undeveloped equilibratory apparatus and lack of strength. Furthermore, the narrow base of steps during these stepping movements is in marked contrast to the wide base adopted in the footwork of the beginning toddler.

One may also speculate as to the role of the plantar reflex in such neonatal stepping movements, since tactual stimulation of the sole of the foot is involved in both these responses. Although the observations of Minkowski (1922) of the plantar reflex during the late fetal period would indicate the establishment of the adult toe flexion pattern at this time, numerous other investigators have reported widely divergent responses in the neonate. Toe extensions are reported as occurring more frequently than toe flexions (Richards and Irwin, 1934) whereas, in another instance, the nature of the response is noted as depending upon the previous posture of the toes so that a posture of flexion will result in extension and vice versa (Sherman and Sherman, 1925). A very exhaustive study of the patterning of the responses to stimulation of the sole of the foot reveals almost 200 different patterns of which the five most frequent were: foot flexion; extension of the toes and foot flexion; extension of the hallux; toes extended, fanning, and foot flexion; and hallux extension and foot flexion (Pratt, 1954).

The grasping reflex has been interpreted by some investigators, as has the Moro response, as a defensive mechanism in terms of the arboreal phylogenetic development of man and, because of its digital character, has sometimes been described as simian. The grasp of the neonate, which involves palm and finger flexion without thumb opposition when the infant is partially or wholly suspended, is considered to be involuntary whereas the adult grasp, with opposing thumb, is voluntary. In terms of behavior sequence, involuntary grasping disappears at about 4 to 6 months of age, after which it is replaced by the adult form of grasping (Pratt, 1954). However, no abrupt change occurs in the grasping sequence as there is some overlapping of the two forms. Careful studies of the neonatal grasping reflex indicate two phases; namely, the closure of the fingers to light pressure upon the palm, and, secondly, the gripping or clinging which is considered to be a proprioceptive response to pull on the finger tendons. A discrepancy in the times of disappearance of closure, in about 16 to 24 weeks, and of proprioceptive gripping or clinging, after 25 weeks, is accounted for by the observation that closure is a specific or limited response whereas gripping or clinging has other movements associated with it (Halverson, 1937).

The length of time that an infant can support its own weight, is often used as a measure of the strength of the grasp. The average length of suspension time with two hands has been found to be 60

seconds with the longest time being 128 seconds (Richter, 1934).
When pulled toward suspension, infants are generally able to support more than 70 percent of their body weight. During the testing
of 97 infants under 24 weeks of age, Halverson (1937) found that 27
were able to support their entire weight in the process of being
pulled to suspension while one infant, 4 weeks old, was able to complete the process with the right hand alone. Age would seem to be a
factor, since the strength of the grasping response was not as great
during the early part of the neonatal period. Furthermore, when
the gripping strength of the infant was measured by means of a
small, sensitive rubber capsule, it was noted that the strength of the
grasp was greatest during the early part of nursing and decreased as
the infant approached satiety (Halverson, 1937). The grasp of the
infant is also recorded as being strongest when the infant is crying
and weakest when it is asleep (Sherman et al., 1936). These results
would certainly indicate that muscular tension, as it is reflected in
the strength of grasp, is dependent, as are so many of the functions
during the neonatal period, upon the physiological condition of
the infant.

Differences have been reported in the grasping strength of the
two hands with the left hand averaging 1765 grams while the right
hand was found to average 1732 grams (Sherman et al., 1936).
Clinging strength has also been noted as being slightly superior in
the left hand (Halverson, 1937). It would appear, therefore, that the
left hand is stronger than the right in the neonate although the reverse tends to be true in the adult where right-handedness is most
common. Studies of handedness in the neonate have involved attempts at assessing the preferential arm motility. In some instances,
no difference has been found in the preferential motility of the arms
(Watson 1919) whereas, in other instances, a significantly greater
degree of motility was observed in the right arm (Stubbs and Irwin,
1933; Valentine and Wagner, 1934). However, such motility did not
appear to be related to later preferential reaching by some of the
same subjects.

Although the neonate does possess a repertory of sensory motor
responses, it is possible that intelligent behavior, as defined by some
investigators of human behavior, must await further maturation.
Irwin (1942) has proposed four criteria for intelligent behavior in

an organism; namely, functional distance receptors, a functional cerebral cortex, an upright posture, and the achievement of symbolical or substitutive behavior. According to this definition, intelligent behavior is impossible in the neonate. However, normative studies of sensory and motor responses at this period are valuable in estimating levels of development and in identifying some pathological neural conditions.

CHAPTER VI

MOTOR BEHAVIOR OF INFANTS

Once the infant has successfully established the physiological transitions after birth necessary in its adaptation to the new environment, the processes of growth and maturation proceed apace in the development of behavior necessary for the continued successful functioning of the organism. The term growth is usually assigned to measurable physical and biological changes in the development of the individual but the definition of maturation leads to a greater divergence of opinion among investigators in the field of child development. Gesell (1933) considers maturation to be the intrinsic regulatory mechanism which preserves the balance and direction of the total pattern of growth while Krogman (1950) defines maturation as a time-linked phase, or process, leading to the ultimate status of maturity of each different structure.

MATURATION AND LEARNING

Although no exact definition of maturation has been universally accepted, the term is most frequently used to describe changes which develop in an orderly fashion without direct influence of known external stimuli but which are almost certainly, in part at least, a product of the interaction of the organism and its environment. With respect to higher organisms it is certainly true that no adaptive function is at its optimum of perfection from the moment of its inception. For example, at a certain stage in the development of the child it becomes possible for him to attempt to walk. Our common expression, learning to walk, recognizes the need for practice to perfect this function.

Investigators in the field of development are frequently confronted with the problem of distinguishing between changes in behavior resulting from the processes of maturation and of learning on the part of the individual. Essential characteristics of maturation are usually listed as: the sudden appearance of new patterns of growth or behavior; the appearance of particular abilities without benefit of previous practice; the consistency of these patterns in different subjects of the same species; the orderly sequence in the manifestation of different patterns; and the gradual course of physical and biological growth toward the attainment of mature status.

A number of studies on lower animals have demonstrated the importance of interaction between the organism and its environment. The technique of restricting function beyond the normal period of inception of a particular behavior characteristic has been employed in a number of these investigations. Spalding (1873) hooded young chicks and kept them from the hen for varying periods of time. Those chicks which had been hooded and kept from the hen for only a day or two would, upon release, run to the hen in response to her call, whereas chicks which had been kept from the hen for a period of ten or more days did not respond to the calls of the hen. These results led Spalding to surmise that the moment of "ripeness" during which the chick can be induced to respond to and follow the hen had been exceeded in the latter instance. Similarly, restraining young swallows beyond the time when they would ordinarily begin to fly indicated varying degrees of efficiency among the birds during their first flight although all were able to fly (Spalding, 1875). Moreover, ten weeks of confinement of young buzzards starting just as they were beginning to feather resulted in a high degree of impairment of flight and balancing ability on the part of the confined birds in comparison with their unrestrained nest mates who were soaring with adult skill by this time. Subsequent observations over a period of several weeks revealed a continued impairment in the flight of the experimental birds which was attributed to their prolonged confinement (Dennis, 1941).

Similar results have been obtained by investigators working with mammals. Introduction of mice into the cages of kittens who have previously never seen a mouse produces remarkably different results with increasing age. If the mouse is introduced for the first time when the kitten is in its second month the change in behavior of the kitten is so marked that kittens may be conceived to kill mice instinctively. This behavior is increasingly difficult to evoke if the the mouse is introduced for the first time at a later age of the kitten (Yerkes and Bloomfield, 1910). More recent experimentation with chimpanzees has carried the period of restriction still further, in some cases completely depriving the animal of any opportunity for the exercise of certain functions over periods of time as long as one year. Permanent impairment results from such experimental deprivation. *Studies have shown that infants exposed to minimal out of rate stimulation of social stimulation, suffered from certain deficits that then were no deleterious effect socially.*

Studies involving restriction of activity in humans do not, in general, reveal such dramatic results as those with animals. Moral considerations prevent investigators from carrying experiments to the extent where serious malfunctioning or atypical behavior will result. Some restriction was involved in a study by Dennis (1935, 1938) in which twin girls were reared from the age of one month to fourteen months under nursery conditions with a minimal amount of motor and social stimulation. When the development of these infants was compared to standard norms, it was found that they were retarded in certain motor achievements beyond the age range for the appearance of these items in normal infants. Social development, however, showed no appreciable difference between the ratings of the twins and standard norms so that customary social stimulation does not appear to be indispensable for normal social behavioral development at this age.

Various cultures often impose restrictions upon the motor activity of infants and these provide a fertile area of exploration without infringing upon the mores of the culture. Such physical restrictions are placed upon infants in the Albanian culture, where babies are bound to small wooden cradles during the first year and are released only for purposes of cleaning. An investigation which rated the Albanian children on the basis of the Viennese infant tests indicated some retardation in motor development on the part of these children, particularly during the third year. Social development, however, was found to be normal in the Albanian children, as could logically be expected since they received the greatest amount of stimulation in this area (Danzinger and Frankl, 1934).

Similar studies of the influences of cradle binding as employed by the Hopi Indians, however, revealed no appreciable degree of difference in motor development in comparison with the norms for American infants (Dennis, 1940). In this instance, as opposed to the more stringent binding restrictions of the Albanians, the Indian infants were allowed varying amounts of freedom from the confines of the cradle. During the first three months of cradle binding, the Hopi child is, except for approximately one hour daily, constantly bound to the cradle. After three months, the number and time duration of the periods of freedom are increased. Currently, more and more Hopi children are being reared with complete freedom of movement and a comparison of 43 of these with 63 Hopi infants who had been reared on cradle boards indicated that the median age of walking for the latter group was 14.98 months while that of the free group was 14.5 months (Dennis and Dennis, 1940). These results were, however, based upon the recollection of parents whose children were from 2 to 6 years of age at the time of this study and there may, therefore, be some question as to the reliability of this information. In general, the results of these studies indicate that the physical restrictions imposed by the Hopi Indians on their infants by cradle binding are within the range that can be tolerated by humans and still result in normal progress. In comparison with the Albanian cradle binding, they also tend to indicate that the amount of motor activity required by the infant for normal development increases throughout the first year.

EFFECTS OF ADDITIONAL PRACTICE ON DEVELOPMENT

Rather than attempting to assess learning by the technique of restricting practice, most investigators in human behavior development have tended to augment normal opportunities by additional practice as a more culturally acceptable method of approaching the problem of differentiating maturation and learning. A very careful study by Gesell and Thompson (1929), using identical twins, of the effects of practice at the threshold age for climbing and cube combining indicated to these investigators that learning appears to be profoundly conditioned by maturation. Starting at 46 weeks of age, Twin T was given 10 minutes of practice and encouragement for 6 days a week in climbing a four tread staircase and in manipulating cubes. The training continued for 6 weeks and was directed towards an expansion of the activities, not just their initiation. During this first training period, Twin C, the control twin, was deprived of stairs and cubes but not restricted in any other way. At the end of the 6 weeks of training, or at 52 weeks, the experimental twin, T, was able to climb the stairs in 10 to 18 seconds. At the same age but with no previous training, the control twin, C, was able to climb the stairs in 40 seconds. However, 2 weeks of training started at 53 weeks and similar to that given to Twin T lowered C's time to 10 to 18 seconds by the end of this particular training period. Neither twin was then trained nor tested until one week later at 56 weeks when the re-test results were:

1st	Trial	Twin T	11.3 sec.
1st	Trial	Twin C	14.8 sec.
2nd	Trial	Twin T	13.8 sec.
2nd	Trial	Twin C	13.9 sec.

On the basis of these results Gesell and Thompson concluded that training does not transcend maturation but that maturation does tend to modify or supplant the results of training.

Furthermore, Gesell and Thompson noted that, although the times for the completion of stair climbing were similar at the end of the experiment, Twin T was admittedly more skillful prior to the inception of Twin C's training period and tended to remain more skillful ten weeks later. Sixteen weeks after the beginning of Twin C's training period, Twin T was still reported as being more agile, less afraid of falling, and walking faster. Twenty-six weeks later Twin T was noted to traverse more ground during play and to be more mobile. McGraw (1946) expresses the opinion that the real issue in the Gesell and Thompson study is not whether practice had any effect on the emergence of the climbing or cube building activities but involves a consideration of the relative effects of practice as associated with the time of introduction of the practice period. Certainly it would appear that the practice sessions were much more effective at the later period when the infant had presumably achieved the degree of maturity necessary for rapid improvement to accrue from such practice.

Similarly, as experimental study of young children trained in cutting with scissors, buttoning, and climbing a ladder showed that, although the experimentally trained group exceeded the non--practice control group in all tests after 12 weeks of practice, the control group was able at a later date with only one week of practice, to achieve the same level of performance as the experimental group (Hilgard, 1932). The greater profit from training within a shorter period of time shown by the control youngsters at a slightly older age led this investigator to conclude that factors other than training contributed to the development of the three skills used in the study. Maturation and practice in related skills were cited as each making partial contributions to the more effective later practice period. It would appear, therefore, that for short term training the period in the maturation of the child at which training is undertaken must receive serious consideration for the achievement of the most effective results from the least amount of practice.

A longitudinal study of fraternal twin boys was undertaken by McGraw (1935) to determine the age at which children will show improvement in various motor activities from practice. The experimental twin, Johnny, was trained in activities in which he was somewhat capable from the time he was 21 days old until the age of 22 months while the control twin, Jimmy, was kept in a crib so that his activities were comparatively restricted. Additional items were added to Johnny's practice repertory as he grew older and was more capable of performing the new activities. During the course of the experiment, the behavior development of the twins was compared to that of a group of 68 children who were also being observed in these same activities. Johnny was advanced in those events in which he had received training while Jimmy fell within the developmental norm range. On the basis of her observations, McGraw concludes that there are critical periods for any given activity when it is most susceptible to modification through repetition of performance. She also points out that phylogenetic activities, (those which every child must acquire in order to function biologically as a human being,) are maturationally fixed and less subject to modification through repetition of performance than are the ontogenetic activities, namely those which an individual may or may not acquire.)

Numerous investigators have stressed the consistency of the sequential order of development of locomotion in infancy (Gesell, 1928; Shirley, 1931, 1933; Bayley, 1935; Ames, 1937; McGraw, 1940a). There would appear to be little modification of the development of bipedal locomotion through practice, nor is there any evidence that practice will have much influence on the subsequent development of the phylogenetic activities of running, jumping, and throwing. With ontogenetic, or culturally influenced, activities such as bicycle riding or roller skating, however, the availability of equipment and the opportunity for practice have a marked influence upon the acquisition of these skills. For example, with training, Johnny was able to roller skate soon after he was able to walk whereas some individuals never achieve this skill throughout their entire lives. Early training does, moreover, seem to have a very definite effect upon the individual's general "rapport" or "feeling" for motor activities. Although later observations of Johnny and Jimmy revealed, on the basis of objective tests, that both were of somewhat equal skill level, Johnny, who had been given the greater opportunity for motor activity during his first two years, still exhibited superior motor coordination and also more assurance in his movements many years after the termination of the experiment than was shown by the previously less active Jimmy (McGraw, 1939b).

SIZE AND PROPORTIONS

The physical growth of the infant with its developmental changes in body proportion has a very definite influence in the motor behavior possibilities available to the infant. For example, the mode of prehension of the infant will be influenced by the size of the child's hand in relation to the size and mobility of the object to be seized. Aside from the problems of strength, it would also seem logical that the large head and small limbs present problems of

both balance and motive power in the achievement of upright
locomotion.

At birth, 1/4 of the body length is taken up by the head with the
ratio of trunk length to lower limb length being approximately 4:3
in the remaining 3/4's of the total body length. During the first half
year the rapid growth is mainly a process of filling out and broaden-
ing with only relatively slight changes in body proportion. While
growth continues to be rapid during the remaining period of infancy, this subsequent growth is marked by increasing changes in
body proportion. The period after the first six months up until
puberty is noted for slow head growth, rapid limb growth and an
intermediate rate of growth in trunk length so that by the end of
two years of age the lower limbs and trunk of the child are approximately equal in length (See Figure 8).

Although the weight of the male exceeds that of the female by 4
percent and the height excess is 2 percent over the female at
birth, the greater maturity of the female is reflected even at the
early age of 8 weeks in the relatively longer lower limbs. The percentage rate of growth does not differ significantly between the sexes
even though the growth increment tends to be larger for the male.
Therefore, it is entirely possible that the slightly longer lower limbs
together with the lesser weight of the female may be a factor, in
addition to greater maturity, in the tendency for females to acquire
skill in upright locomotion before males.

Since ponderal growth in infancy follows the general course of
growth in height, pediatricians rely on weight gain as evidence of
adequate nutrition. Indications are that infants from poorer homes
are shorter and weigh less than those from economically adequate
homes (Bakwin and Bakwin, 1931), while the retardation in bodily
dimensions which accompanies retardation in weight is greater for
the transverse than for the vertical dimensions. This results in the
youngsters from poorer homes being comparatively more linear than
those from economically adequate homes. In instances where proper
care is given to infants from poorer homes in a clinic the height and
weight is raised and a change also occurs in the relative body proportions so as to conform with the norms of a control group (Bakwin and Bakwin, 1936). Studies indicate that there is no difference
in size between Negro and white infants in similar economic circumstances (Bakwin and Patrick, 1944). Nor does there appear to

be any evidence showing racial differences between Negroes and whites in rate of growth (Scott et al., 1950).

DEVELOPMENT OF UPRIGHT LOCOMOTION

During the first two years of postnatal life, striking progress is made by the comparatively helpless newborn infant in its development. Within this short period of time, the infant becomes a young child who has assumed an erect posture and is capable of bipedal locomotion. At the same time, the upper extremities have also been undergoing rapid developmental changes so that by the end of this period the child has attained manual dexterity in reaching, grasping, and fine manipulation. While, for purposes of discussion, it is more convenient to treat locomotor and prehensive development separately, it should be remembered that these developmental processes are occurring simultaneously although there may be variations within any individual with respect to either as compared to developmental norms.

Studies of the development of erect posture and bipedal locomotion in the human infant have centered around the identification of phases, the order of appearance of phases, and the factors associated with the time of onset of these phases. Since different investigators have, in some instances, identified different phases, there are naturally some slight discrepancies in time sequences. Moreover, observations tend to be based upon averages of performance of a number of children so that it is also possible that all phases do not occur in all children nor that their duration is the same for all children.

Although listing a greater number of activities as indicative of locomotor development, Shirley (1931b) combines them into five main stages which are indicative of the progressive phases necessary for the achievement of upright posture, of walking, and of a temporary means of locomotion, usually creeping, until bipedal locomotion is established. These stages, together with their inclusive activities, are listed in Table 1.

In Table 1, the activities marked with an asterisk (*) indicate those which Shirley believes mark progression in the development of upright posture while those marked with an accent mark (') are indicative of progression in the attainment of bipedal locomotion.

Table I
Development of Locomotion†

Stage	Time of onset	Activity
1. Postural control of upper body.	Before 20 weeks	Chin up* Chest up* Stepping' Sit on lap*
2. Postural control of entire trunk and undirected activity.	25 to 31 weeks	Sit alone momentarily* Knee push or swim Rolling Stand with help' Sit alone 1 minute
3. Active efforts at locomotion.	37 to 39.5 weeks	Some progress on stomach Scoot backward
4. Locomotion by creeping.	42 to 47 weeks	Stand holding to furniture* Creep Walk when led' Pull to stand*
5. Postural control and coordination for walking.	62 to 64 weeks	Stand alone' Walk alone'

---

† Adapted from M. M. Shirley, *The First Two Years. A Study of Twenty-five Babies. Volume 1. Postural and Locomotor Development.* Minneapolis: University of Minnesota Press, 1931. By permission of the publisher.

According to this investigator, the unmarked activities are those employed by the child to provide a temporary means of locomotion and merely overlap the other two categories without adding to their development other than by the incidental increase in strength resulting from such activity.

A listing of 23 stages in the development of behavior eventuating in standing and walking has been divided into activities which are considered to be either flexor- or extensor-dominated by Gesell and Ames (1940). Here all stages are believed to exhibit the slow but sure sequence of postural transformations necessary for the final achievement of upright posture and locomotion, with none of the stages being considered as capable of dismissal on the basis of their possi-

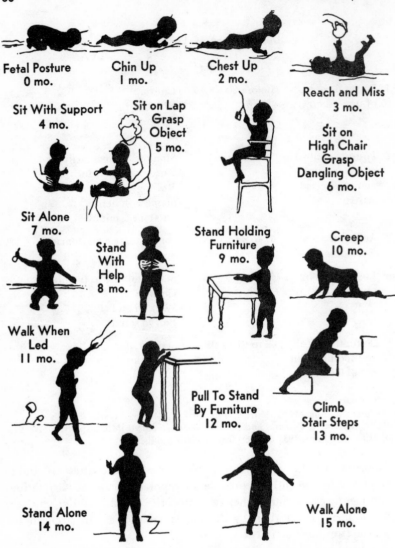

Fetal Posture
0 mo.

Chin Up
1 mo.

Chest Up
2 mo.

Reach and Miss
3 mo.

Sit With Support
4 mo.

Sit on Lap
Grasp
Object
5 mo.

Sit on
High Chair
Grasp
Dangling Object
6 mo.

Sit Alone
7 mo.

Stand
With
Help
8 mo.

Stand Holding
Furniture
9 mo.

Creep
10 mo.

Walk When
Led
11 mo.

Pull To Stand
By Furniture
12 mo.

Climb
Stair Steps
13 mo.

Stand Alone
14 mo.

Walk Alone
15 mo.

Figure 10.   Developmental sequence in bipedal locomotion. (From M. M. Shirley, **The First Two Years. A Study of Twenty-five Babies. Volume II. Intellectual Development.** Minneapolis: University of Minnesota Press, 1933. By permission of the publisher.)

ble recapitulatory or vestigial nature. Compression of these 23 stages into four cycles, each comprised of what is considered to be a "continuum of closely related stages," illustrate, to some extent, the fluctuations in dominance between extensors and flexors as well as the integration of unilateral, bilateral, and crossed lateral movements into more complex movements. In general, upright locomotion eventually involves a permanent preponderance of extensor action while the most mature expression of flexor dominance occurs in creeping.

1. In the first cycle (stages 1-10, covering the first 29 weeks of life) the dominant pattern of bilateral flexion of arms and legs which is present at birth gradually gives way to more mature unilateral flexion of the extremities. During this cycle the trunk remains in contact with the supporting surface, although the extremities are used with limited success for circular locomotion.

2. During the second cycle (stages 11-19, the 30th through the 42nd week) the infant is able to elevate the trunk above the table surface. This requires a temporary reversion of the arms to the more elemental position of bilateral flexion. The predominate motor patterns of this cycle include bilateral extension of arms and bilateral extension and flexion of the legs as observed in the backward crawl, the low creep, the high creep and rocking. In Stage 19 the creep involves a high level of movement with rather involved coordinations, for not only is there alternate extension of the arms and alternate flexion of the legs, but these movements occur with the members of the opposite side moving alternately.

3. The third cycle (stages 21a and 21b, the 49th through 56th week) entails a temporary reversion to an immobile bilateral extension in maintaining the plantigrade stance. Shortly thereafter, arms and legs extend forward alternately in plantigrade progression, the right arm and leg moving simultaneously.

4. The fourth cycle (stages 22 and 23, the 50th through 60th week) finds the infant capable of full trunk extension and assuming an upright posture. Walking follows as the arms and legs extend bilaterally, but with the movements occurring alternately.*

From the foregoing excerpt and from Figure 11, partial reversion at intervals to a less mature pattern is indicated, so that total pro-

---

* From G. L. Rarick, *Motor Development During Infancy and Childhood.* Madison, Wis.: University of Wisconsin, 1954. By permission of the author.

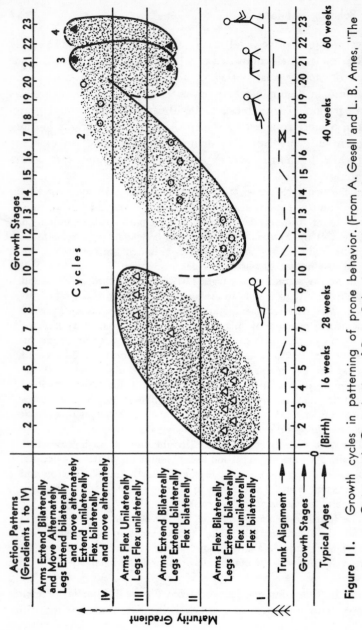

Figure 11. Growth cycles in patterning of prone behavior. (From A. Gesell and L. B. Ames, "The Ontogenetic Organization of Prone Behavior in Human Infancy." **J. Genet. Psychol.,** 56: 247-263, 1940. By permission of the publisher, The Journal Press.)

90

gression towards a more mature state is of a spiral nature (Gesell, 1954). Such an interpretation is not forthcoming from other investigators, however, and seeming "delays" or "reversions" are explained in terms of the development of functional equilibrium. The infant must be able to control its body in any new postural alignments in a static position before it can undertake the shifting postural sets which accompany a new skill (Shirley, 1931). In short, mastery of upright posture and locomotion depends upon the functional development of equilibrium, which has a cephalic status in the vestibular apparatus and a caudal status with the foot as the final fulcrum of locomotion. With each new postural alignment, then, cerebral adjustments involving both equilibrium and neuromuscular responses would be required in a static posture before control could be expected in more complicated dynamic movements.

Variations in the time of onset of various phases of locomotion are most clearly indicated in a comparison of the median ages at which both Shirley and Bayley observed such motor activity in 25 and 61 infants respectively (Bayley, 1935). As well as pointing up variations in performance ages, Figure 12 also indicates that the development of children in California, the site of Bayley's study, tends to be generally more advanced than that of the children of Minnesota where Shirley's records were obtained.

The study of 25 children from birth to two years of age by Shirley (1931) also revealed additional trends in locomotor behavior other than the sequential developmental phases which are considered to be typical of locomotor behavior in the attainment of upright posture and walking. As soon as the child is able to walk alone, he is able to increase his speed rapidly and, in the process of doing so, also increases the length of step, decreases the width of the step and gradually reduces the angle at which the leg is raised. Increasing ability of the child to maintain balance during upright locomotion is reflected by decreased use of the arms for balance and the reduction of the base of support involved in the decrease in the width of the step together with a reduction in the degree of toeing out of the foot.

Although Shirley did not find any definite relationship between her measures of motor development and anatomical and physiological measurements of the child, Norval (1947) noted that, for new-

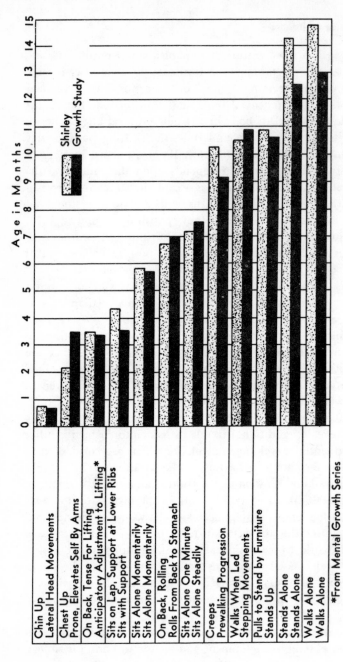

Figure 12. Comparison of data from Shirley and from California Infant Growth Study on median age of first passing certain motor items. (From Nancy Bayley, "The Development of Motor Abilities during the First Three Years." **Monogr. Soc. Res. Child Develpm.**, 1(1):1-26, 1935. By permission of the author and publisher.)

*From Mental Growth Series

born infants of the same weight, a difference of one inch in length tends to indicate that the longer child will, on the average, walk 22 days earlier than the shorter child. Sex difference is commonly noted to favor females in the earlier onset of walking, but Nicolson and Hanley (1953) report the mean age for walking of 114 boys to be 13.4 months while that for 123 girls was 13.6 months. Certainly physique, heredity, and environment play a definite part in the time of onset of upright posture and walking. Small boned and muscular infants have been noted as tending to walk earlier than those who are short, rotund, and exceedingly heavy while an association has also been made between early skill in walking and such factors as good muscular strength and interest in gross motor play (Shirley, 1931).

PREHENSION DEVELOPMENT

Although the newborn infant will grasp an object of appropriate size that is placed in the palm, prehensive activity involving eye-hand coordination must await the attainment of control of the oculomotor muscles. Infants will take little notice of a cube or similar sized object placed within reach nor make any effort to reach them before 16 weeks of age. After this time, the sight of objects will result in arm activation but not reaching as such. By the time the youngster is 20 weeks old, the "corralling" action of both arms and hands working together has developed to the extent where the infant begins to consistently attain the object rather than pushing it out of reach through lack of control when contact is made. After the object has been corralled, it is often picked up in one hand by a palm grasp in which the thumb and fingers retain the object against the palm of the hand. Four weeks later prehension involves the approaching and grasping of an object with one hand; however, such reaching is composed of the distinct movements of raising the hand, a circuitous thrusting forward of the hand, and then a final lowering of the hand to grasp the object. By approximately the 40th week, reaching and grasping have become coordinated into a single, continuous movement (Halverson, 1931; Gesell and Ilg, 1946).

The use of the hand in grasping objects undergoes a change from the thumb and finger palm grasp of early prehension to the mature pincer-like movement of the thumb against the forefinger. This development involves an ulnar-radial shift in the positioning of the grasped object that is closely associated with the increased use of thumb opposition. While the crude palmar grasp which tends to favor the ulnar aspect of the palm is evident at 20 weeks, there is a definite trend towards preference for the radial area of the palm for grasping and manipulating objects by 28 weeks. With the development of the thumb-index finger approach to objects which require precise prehension by the end of the first year, the ulnar-radial shift becomes complete. Figure 13, based upon cinematographic records, illustrates this progressive development of grasping.

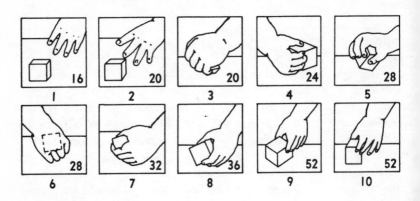

Figure 13.   Developmental progression in grasping. (From H. M. Halverson, "An Experimental Study of Prehension in Infants by Means of Systematic Cinema Records." **Genet. Psychol. Monogr.,** 10:107-286, 1931. By permission of the publisher, The Journal Press.)

The complexity of the processes inherent in the developmental progression of voluntary reaching and grasping is indicated by the six component coordinate acts that Landreth (1958) believes to be involved in the development of prehension. The first of these is the transition from visually locating an object to attempting to reach for the object. Other transitions involve: (2) simple eye-hand coordination, to progressive independence of visual effort with its ultimate expression in activities such as piano playing and typing; (3) initial maximal involvement of body musculature to a minimum involvement and greater economy of effort; (4) proximal large muscle activity of the arms and shoulders to distal fine muscle activity of the fingers; (5) early crude raking movements in manipulating objects with the hands to the later pincer-like precision of control with the opposing thumb and forefinger; and (6) initial bilateral reaching and manipulation to ultimate use of the preferred hand.

Neural development undoubtedly plays a primary role in the acquisition and development of all motor skills, including prehension, and, in the case of those activities which are not reflex in nature. would appear to precede such motor development by a considerable period of time. The greatest cortical development of the newborn infant has been found to be in the area of the anterior central gyrus which mediates movements of the neck and shoulders while the greatest change that occurs by the time the infant is one month old is noted to be in the region of the hand of the motor area of the gyrus centralis (Conel, 1939, 1941).

In addition to the increasing evidences of coordination and of precision of movement which reflect improvements in neuromuscular functioning, the number of objects which the infant handles adds a further measure to the complexity of manual dexterity and as such provides an overt indicator of neuromuscular functioning and maturation. A study of 178 infants in which such objects as a block, rattle, ball, steel tape measure, metal tube, and tongue depressor were handed to the children indicated that approximately 80 percent of infants would accept and hold one object at 5 months, two objects at 8 months, and three objects at 11½ months (Lippman, 1927) It is quite obvious that the items in this particular study differ in size and shape, so that, although it does indicate increased complexity of manual dexterity as measured by the number of objects handled, caution should be exercised in accepting the figures as being exact with respect to both the number of objects and the age placement. Such caution is based upon the factors of the size of the child's hand and the size. shape, and texture of the objects, which will affect the child's mode of prehension and the number of objects he may successfully handle (McGraw, 1946)

PREFERENTIAL HANDEDNESS

The development of preferred handedness has been of concern to numerous investigators on a purely developmental basis, as it is related to cultural influences, and as a possible factor in the development of speech or reading problems. The earliest postnatal manifestation of hand preference is believed, by some investigators, to be the tonic neck reflex. However, it has been noted that, during the first three months, ⅓ of infants consistently assume a right tonic neck reflex while an equal number adopt the left tonic neck reflex with the remaining ⅓ using either a right or left posture in a somewhat ambivalent manner. These ratios provide somewhat different values than are actually reported for right and left handed preference so that some investigators are reluctant to accept handedness as an index of physiologic unilaterality. It has, however, been found that a strong infantile left tonic neck reflex is correlated with emphatic constitutional left handedness (Gesell, 1954).

During infancy and well into childhood, there is a considerable interchanging of the use of either hand and of both hands until unilateral dominance is eventually achieved or, as in some instances, the individual has developed a higher degree of ambidexterity than is usually attained by individuals who are classified as unilaterally dominant. In one study of the development of handedness, contact with the object by the infant of 16 to 20 weeks was found to be unilateral and with the left hand. At 24 weeks, contact was bilateral while four weeks later it was unilateral with contact usually being made with the right hand. By 32 weeks, it was again bilateral after which time unilateral dominance alternated from right to left hand for the remainder of the first year. The right hand again dominated between the 52nd and 56th weeks followed by considerable interchangeability by 80 weeks. At two years, the right hand was in ascendency but there was again bilaterality between 2½ and 4 years. Following this, the right hand continued to become increasingly dominant (Gesell and Ames, 1947). Clearly there is a great deal of interchangeability of hand preference in most infants but great individual differences exist in the amount of such interchangeability and in its patterning. For example, another study indicates that infants will accept objects in the right hand 50 percent of the time at 4½ months whereas the previously cited observations of Gesell and Ames indicate that this is a period in which the left hand is preferred (Lippman, 1927).

In a study of 40 nursery school children who were tested on hand preference in spinning a top, spooning sand, shaking a rattle, and hammering a block, Updegraff (1932) placed 35 in a right hand preference category while the remaining 5 were considered to be predominantly left handed. Examination of these unilateral dominance classifications, however, revealed that use was made of the right hand between 50 to 97 percent of the time by those placed in the right handed category while the percentage use of the left hand by the children considered to be left handed was 55 to 85. Similar studies of 44 nursery school children by Hildreth (1948, 1949) revealed that children tend to be more right handed and more consistent in their use of this hand in taught activities such as drawing with a crayon, eating with implements, and throwing a ball than they are in the untaught activities such as eating with their fingers. Such results certainly support the position that children of this age are not exclusively right or left handed.

Right handedness is not only found to be more common in learned activities but also increases with age in our culture. Eighty to ninety percent of nursery school and kindergarten children are right handed, while among adults the percentage ranges from 95 to 97 (Landreth, 1958). However, boys, who tend to be less responsive to and/or less subjected to as much social training as girls, are more often left handed than the opposite sex. Moreover, retarded children and mental defectives, who are also less responsive to social training, have twice as great an incidence of left handedness as normal children. The changing mores of our culture and increase in knowledge are creating a greater leniency on the part of the public to left hand preference resulting in a current increase in the proportion of left handed children. Whether this increase will ever establish the approximate 50-50 percentage base that is found in eyedness is questionable however. Even in primitive societies where little attention is given to handedness the proportion still favors right handedness while exposure to a classroom situation markedly tips the scales in favor of the right hand. For example, 1047 African primary school children, aged 6 to 13 years, were tested with three tests of handedness, namely, unscrewing the cap on a bottle, cutting out a paper circle with scissors, and erasing a word, and only .5 percent of the children were found to be left handed (Verhaegen and Ntumba, 1964).

It would appear, therefore, that hand preference is, to a great extent, culturally conditioned and would seem to have been so historically. A left handed person would have been at a considerable disadvantage in the not too distant past when swords were worn on the left side. There is still a hold-over of this custom in the European positioning of the woman in relation to her male escort. Regardless of the position of the gutter, which has affected such social niceties in other areas, the female is always to the right of the male. This was to prevent the man's sword from becoming entangled in the voluminous female skirts.

Since our culture is oriented to favor right handedness, some pressure is usually exerted upon children to change from preferential use of the left hand to that of the right. Six prognostic indicators for a favorable transfer of handedness have been suggested by Hildreth (1950). These should be considered so as to avoid the possibility of conflict with any innate disposition toward hand preference. They are as follows: (1) the child should be under six years of age and (2) use both hands interchangeably with (3) the handedness index being bilateral. In addition, the child must be (4) above average in intelligence and (5) be agreeable to the change with the (6) resulting trial period showing no difficulty in transition from the left hand to the right.

The period of late infancy and early childhood is the time in which mental integration, manual lateral dominance, and speech are all in a period of rapid development. Thus it is entirely possible that a feeling of insecurity with respect to manual dexterity may transfer to speech (Landreth, 1958). Whether there is actually a cause and effect relationship here is not clear, however. It has been observed that some left handed children have begun to stutter when attempts were made to change their hand preference. There are more stutterers among left handed children and childern who are inconsistent in their handedness than among right handed children. There is also a greater incidence of stuttering among boys than among girls. However, stutterers frequently exhibit other behavior difficulties, not necessarily inconsistent handedness. It is quite possible that both types of problems stem from some more deep-seated cause and that the apparent relationship between them is due to their simultaneous occurrence.

OTHER ASPECTS OF GROWTH AND BEHAVIOR

It is very obvious from the foregoing that all aspects of the development of the child are interrelated and cannot be broken into separate entities. Furthermore, there is a patterning to this whole development that is reflected in the separate facets that have been outlined. McGraw (1939a) holds that there are four outstanding periods which may be classified roughly in terms of the type of development taking place during the first two years. The first period, of approximately four months, is identified by a marked diminution of the rhythmical and atavistic reflexes which are characteristic of the newborn. The next four to eight months, or second period, is typified by the development of voluntary movements in the superior spinal region and the comparative reduction of activity in the region of the pelvic girdle and lower extremities. The third period, which extends through the fourteenth month, is marked by the increasing control of activities in the lower spinal region and the fourth period, which covers the remaining ten months, is characterized by the rapid development of conditional and symbolic associational processes including langauge.

Other investigators have identified slightly different aspects and placed slightly different emphases on them but the general trends observed in behavior development tend to be very similar. Gesell makes this statement:

In the first quarter (4-16 weeks) of the first year the infant gains control of his twelve oculomotor muscles.

In the second quarter (16-28 weeks) he comes in command of the muscles which support his head and move his arms. He reaches for things.

In the third quarter (28-40 weeks) he gains command of his trunk and hands. He sits. He grasps, transfers, and manipulates objects.

In the fourth quarter (40-52 weeks) he extends command to his legs and feet; to his forefinger and thumb. He pokes and plucks. He stands upright.

In the second year he walks and runs; articulates words and phrases; acquires bowel and bladder control; attains a rudimentary sense of personal identity and of personal possession.*

Behavior development during infancy can be correlated fairly well with neurological development. The prominence of the atavistic Moro, grasping, and swimming reflexes indicates that subcortical control of movements is at its maximum toward the end of the first month. After this time there is a progressive decline in these subcortical movements attributed to the onset of cortical inhibition. Later cortical control is first observed in the muscles of the upper body before it appears in the region of the pelvis and lower extremities and typifies the cephalo-caudal principle of developmental direction. The inception of cortical control in a given activity is believed to be marked by staccato and poorly coordinated movements, while further neuromuscular development and cortical control is reflected by an increasing integration of movements rather than actual changes in motor pattern (McGraw, 1941a). The principle of developmental direction explains the cyclic, or spiral, nature of the development of upright progression in terms of successive cephalo-caudal sweeps of development in response to the ascending levels of neural organization appropriate to a certain period (Gesell, 1954).

In addition to the principle of developmental direction, both cephalo-caudal and proximo-distal, which has been a recurring feature of this presentation, other developmental principles have been stated as vital to the functional unity of the human organism. Though the primitive modes of locomotion, such as pivoting, rolling, forward and backward crawl, rocking, creep-crawl, creeping, and cruising, may suggest recapitulation, they should, according to Gesell (1954), be mainly regarded as functional expressions of necessary, though transient, stages in the organization of the neuromotor system. Such organization involves the most fundamental component of muscular movement; namely, the functional relationship between flexion and extension in the counteraction of antagonistic muscles.

---

* From A. Gesell, "The Ontogenesis of Infant Behavior." In L. Carmichael, (Editor). *Manual of Child Psychology.* New York: John Wiley & Sons, Inc., 1954. By permission of the publisher.

Gesell, therefore, believes that a principle of reciprocal interweaving is one of the biological determinants of development. Neurologically, it involves the intricate interweaving of the neural mechanisms of opposing muscle systems into a reciprocal and increasingly mature relationship.

From the discussion of hand preference, it would seem that inconsistency and instability of manual lateral dominance may be reflected in other behavioral areas. To Gesell (1954), hand preference is only one aspect of the principle of functional asymmetry which, in itself, is a special inflection of the principle of reciprocal interweaving. He believes that an asymmetrical focalization of motor set is essential to effective attentional adjustments and that unidexterity of eye, hand, or foot is not so much a representation of absolute skill difference as it is a predilection for stabilized psychomotor orientations.

Additional principles, namely, individuating maturation and self-regulatory fluctuation, are also believed to define vital aspects of growth and behavior. The principle of individuating maturation encompasses the mechanism by which the behavioral organism achieves its species characteristicness, and at the same time makes specific adaptations to its environmental field. For example, the sequential patterning of the behavioral activities terminating in the acquisition of upright locomotion is determined by intrinsic factors and, as such, is species characteristic. However, the minor deviations in technique in the sequential patterning may be accounted for by varying hereditary backgrounds and the interaction of the child's particular intrinsic genetic inheritance with the particular environment and, as such, are a manifestation of the individuating aspects of maturation (Gesell, 1954).

The principle of self-regulatory fluctuation is indicative of the tendency of some behavioral traits to oscillate between two self-limiting poles during their progressive movement toward maturity and stability. It may be recalled that the heart and respiratory rate in the neonate are higher at the resting level and greater in range than in the adult, with progress towards the mature state being marked by a decrease in both the resting frequency and the range during maximal and minimal effort and excitation. Gesell (1954) cites the fluctuating reduction from 19 hours sleep required by the infant during the fourth week to 13 hours in the fortieth week as being indicative of such self-regulatory fluctuation (Figure 14). Certainly the modern emphasis in physiology on the importance of homeostasis would support the importance of this principle in the functioning of human beings.

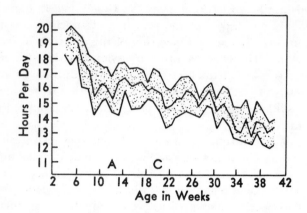

Figure 14.   Child J. Sleep chart from 4 to 40 weeks. (From A. Gesell and F. L. Ilg, **The Feeding Behavior of Infants: A Pediatric Approach to the Mental Hygiene of Early Life.** Philadelphia: J. B. Lippincott Co., 1937. By permission of the publisher.)

As each child moves at his own rate and in his own way through these processes of human development each stimulus and each response expand to some extent his capacities. The important interrelationship of function to structure indicates the vital need for all types of sensory-motor activity. There is wide-spread recognition today of the essential role of early motor experiences as a basis for perceptual and, subsequently, symbolic generalizations. Certainly, then, infancy and childhood should be made particularly rich in all types of motor exploratory opportunities.

CHAPTER VII

MOTOR BEHAVIOR IN EARLY CHILDHOOD

The period of early childhood is usually considered to encompass the age range of 2 to 6 years. Although some investigators have placed the beginning of childhood at 18 months as this is the average age of independent walking, the variations among individuals are great and at no time is there a clear-cut break in human growth characteristics. Therefore, the figure of 2 years is just as acceptable a division between infancy and early childhood and is more frequently used as it lends itself to age comparisons more readily. Furthermore, at about 2 years of age, the relative rate of growth of the child tends to level off in comparison with the rapid growth prior to this time (Figure 15).

PHYSICAL GROWTH

Although gains in height and weight progress at fairly uniform rates during the period of early childhood, the rate of gain in height is nearly twice that in weight. The lower limbs grow rapidly

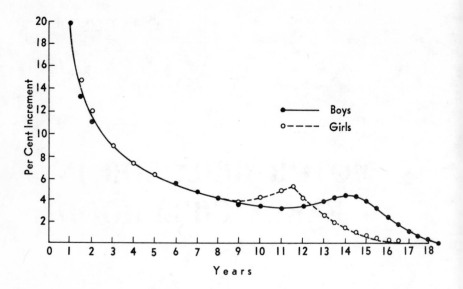

in proportion to the trunk length but neither shoulder nor pelvic
breadth increase rapidly, so that the total configurational change
during childhood is toward a more rectilinear and relatively flat
bodied child (See Figure 8). The male tends to be somewhat taller
and heavier at all ages, but the proportional rate of growth remains
similar for both sexes during this period. Girls maintain their
relatively longer leg length in comparison to stem length until the
end of early childhood. During this period also there is no difference between the sexes with respect to the ratio of shoulder breadth
to pelvic breadth although the measurements for males are slightly
larger than for females.

The proportional increases in bone, muscle, and fat that occur
at this time do not parallel the distribution of these tissues during
either infancy or adulthood. The rate of height gain and the rapid

ossification of the bones indicate that bone tissue plays a significant role in weight increase. The proportion of muscle tissue remains fairly constant at 25 percent until the beginning of the fifth year when 75 percent of the gain in weight is attributed to muscle tissue. First bone and then muscle tissue make their gains at the expense of a reduced rate of gain in fatty tissue. Subcutaneous tissue measurements, before 6 years of age, show a similar pattern for both sexes (Boynton, 1936). The more rapid increase in muscle tissue during the fifth year makes available a larger potential of effective muscular energy for movement in the expanding number of physical activities of the child.

GENERAL DEVELOPMENT

With the start of walking, the world of the child expands rapidly. Quite literally he goes anywhere and everywhere paths are open to him. Since he has increasing amounts of energy available as he grows older and much of this energy is directed into gross motor activity, he needs a safe and, if possible, spacious place to play. In the years from 2 to 6, all of the usual locomotor patterns are perfected and a variety of eye-hand coordinations are learned. The latter are more dependent upon opportunity than the former and are almost certainly more influenced by instruction and encouragement. The child will walk and run, for example, push furniture about and climb onto it in the ordinary course of development. He does not learn to catch or bounce balls nor to strike or bat them without help.

The child usually begins to speak as well as to walk in his second year and, by the age of 2, has a mean vocabulary of 29.1 different words. His comprehension of the meaning of what others are saying increases rapidly, as does his vocabulary (Terman and Merrill, 1937). At 3 years, he has acquired, on the average, a vocabulary of 62.8; at 4 years, 92.6; and at 5½ years, 99.5 words (McCarthy, 1930). The gain in new words is not linear but is greatest during the period 2 to 3 years. This coincides with the beginning of walking. A limited correlation of .39 had been found between the onset of talking and that of walking (Bayley, 1935). To Landreth (1958), these observations suggest that children are ready to make gains in both speech and walking at the same time but do so at the expense of each other, so that the motor skill of upright progression would appear to take precedence over, or develop at the expense of, speech during the period from 15 to 18 months. She also believes that further support is given to the theory of generalized conflict between motor skills and language by the observed sex differences in favor of language in girls and of motor skills in boys.

The manipulative activity of the young child is as constant and all encompassing as time and circumstances will permit. He wants to touch, feel, pick up, carry, and play with every object on which he can get his hands. Through his continuous explorations of both space and things he learns the nature of objects, of space, and to some extent of himself.

The critical nature of early childhood as a period of acquiring motor skills has been stressed by a number of investigators (Hurlock, 1953; Rarick, 1954). Overprotection may hamper a child's motor development by instilling fear in the child of possible bodily harm or by preventing practice during the maturation of particular abilities. Later on, the child may be unable to participate satisfactorily with his peers because of this deficiency or retardation. Such an effect may snowball in that the child's inability to play on equal terms with others further limits his opportunities for practice and so he falls still further behind.

The need for ample opportunity and acceptable means for children to exercise their emerging motor skills is illustrated through an experiment by Johnson (1935). The social behavior of nursery school children was compared with the behavior of the same children after one-half of the equipment had been removed from the playground. A significant increase occurred in the amount of asocial play and physical assault among the children in the more barren surroundings. To Landreth (1958), such results suggested that the children solved the problem of equipment shortage for exercising their newly acquired and developing motor skills by using each other. She strongly recommends that the motor developmental aspect of the child not be neglected at this age level but be encouraged and enhanced as much as possible.

The significant role of motor skills in social development, even at these very early ages, should be noted. The child gains approval from his parents as he learns to do things for himself. His early contacts with other children are frequently through parallel and manipulative play in which objects may circulate among the group. By the fourth year he wants to be with others and to share more vigorous activities. Special skills become important. There would appear to be a reciprocal action between the motor behavior of a child and his emotional responses in that activity promotes a child's well-being and this, in turn, coupled with success in the performance of the activity, leads to expansive action on the part of the child (Landreth, 1958). This reciprocal action between motor behavior and pleasurable feeling is illustrated in reports of numerous investigations that the young child tends to repeat his most recently acquired or developing motor skills. Further, the most frequent cause of smiling in children from 18 to 48 months is their own activity (Ames, 1949). This reaction is not confined to young children, certainly, since many adults experience exhilaration and expansiveness after successfully performing a challenging motor activity.

It will be of interest to study in some detail the development of specific motor patterns in early childhood.

WALKING

The relatively slower rate of growth during the period of early childhood, coupled with the changes in bodily proportions, results in conditions that are increasingly conducive to the development of skill in the recently acquired activity of upright, bipedal locomotion. The child's eagerness to increase his facility in this activity and his contacts with his resultant constantly expanding environment are marked by determination and persistence despite many a tumble and bump.

The pattern of walking undergoes a transition from the first, hesitant, full sole steps with feet widely spread apart to the adult style of walking with a smooth, easy transition of weight in a heel-toe progression from one foot to the other. The rate of walking tends to stabilize at approximately 170 steps per minute between the ages of 18 months and 2 years while, in comparison, the range of steps for four briskly walking adults has been found to be 140 to 145 steps. Of course, adults have a much greater length of stride so that over the same period of time the 2-year-old child, even with a higher step rate, covers only a little more than half the distance traversed by an adult. Since the rate of stride does not increase as rapidly as the amount of distance covered within any period of time, the length of stride must increase from the age of 18 months to 2 years to account for the noted increase in traversed distance (Shirley, 1931).

Along with the increase in the length of stride and the development of a relatively consistent step rate, there is a changing pattern in the use of the foot. During the early stages of walking, out toeing is typical but is gradually replaced by a straighter placement of the foot so that foot alignment in the line of progression is fairly common by the 18th month. Although the length and width of the step become quite uniform between the 20th and 22nd months, the stride of the child is still jerky because of the continued use of the full sole step. However, by the age of 2 years, and in some instances sooner, the transfer of weight from the heel to the toe of the foot upon contacting the ground results in a much smoother walk. By the time the child is 3 years old, walking has become so automatic that little attention needs to be given to it even when the walking surface is slightly uneven. The 3-year-old has developed a good deal of uniformity of length, height, and width of step with heel-toe weight transfer being well established and a certain amount of individuality beginning to appear in the manner in which the child carries his head and trunk. Around the age of 4 years, the child has almost achieved an adult style of walking in his easy, swinging, rhythmical stride and in the smoother transfer of weight in traversing both a straight line or in turning a sharp corner so that the act of walking is now a graceful movement. The use of the foot as both a source of propulsive power and as a rocker to receive and support the body weight has almost approached the adult level of coordination. Although there is great variation among children in the age of accomplishment of mature methods of upright locomotion, in general, it is not until approximately 3 years after the first step is taken, or at around 50 months, that the art of walking may be considered to be perfected in the child (Rarick, 1954).

The problems associated with the acquisition of walking skills revolve largely around the building up of sufficient strength to support the weight of the body temporarily on one leg and the development of the finely adjusted balance mechanisms required for upright locomotion. The wide base of support and the out-stretched arms coupled with the uneven, jerky steps of the beginning walker, often more appropriately called the toddler, is indicative of the struggle with the force of gravity. Even at 2 years of age when some facility in walking and running has been achieved, the child is still only able to maintain his balance on one foot for a very few seconds. Increasing facility in the maintenance of balance is reflected in the ability of the child to walk in a straight line in a given direction. The toddler tends to weave about in progressing from one point to the next with the ability to walk in a straight line in a given direction not being established until the average age of 31.3 months according to one study (Bayley, 1935). In another instance, only one-half of the children tested were able to walk a one inch wide line for a distance of 10 feet without stepping off at the age of 37 months (Wellman, 1937). Greater balance difficulties are presented by the task of walking a circular path, for one-half of a group of children tested were not able to master a circle of 21½ feet without any step-offs until the age of 45 months (Wellman, 1937).

VARIATIONS IN WALKING PATTERNS

It is not surprising that other locomotor activities also require, as does walking, a sufficient degree of strength and the development of the necessary sensory-motor balance mechanisms in addition to the new neuromotor coordinations necessary for successful performance in the new activity. A new activity radically different from the skills already achieved by the child would necessitate tremendous adjustments in these areas. Therefore, it is not surprising that variations of the original basic walking or creeping patterns are gradually established. However, the desire for experimenting with new modes of achieving locomotion is very great during infancy and early childhood, as evidenced by the wide variety of form in the basic modes of prone and upright locomotion. The constant quest for control of the body by children is reflected in the variations of walking achieved very shortly after the establishment of upright locomotion. Walking sideways has been noted to occur at the average age of 16.5 months, walking backwards at 16.9 months, while the more complicated feat of walking on tip-toes is not normally attempted until after 30 months of age (Bayley, 1935). Furthermore, anyone who has ever watched young children at play has seen them pivoting around and around until they become so dizzy they can hardly stand especially upon a soft, grassy surface where a tumble is such fun that it is usually the climax of such activity.

RUNNING

Since the basic limb movements in running are similar to those in walking, little adjustment is required with respect to neuro-muscular patterning but this mechanism must be capable of adjusting to the increased tempo of the run with its quicker inter-action of agonists and antagonists in a coordinated fashion. Strength must also be greater to propel the body off the ground for a short period of time and better balance is required to receive the weight of the body on one foot after its momentary free flight through the air between the steps of the run.

The early type of run which many children adopt at approxi-mately 18 months of age is not a true run but rather a modified walk as there is no period at which the body is not supported by one foot. As heel-toe progression has not become established at this time and the walk itself is stiff legged, the modified run is performed on the entire sole of the foot with the lower limbs being relatively stiff so that the movement is jarring and has an uneven length of stride. The child achieves a smoother stride and run between the ages of two and three but is still lacking control in the ability to stop or turn quickly. Continuing improvement in the power and form of the run results in the gradual accomplish-ment of control over starting, stopping, and turning by the ages of 4 to 5 years. Between the ages of 5 to 6, skill in running has advanced to the level where the adult manner of running is rea-sonably well established and the child is now able to use his run-ning skill effectively in his play activities.

CLIMBING

At about the same time that an infant is learning to creep, he also begins to pull himself up onto his feet so that, with the establishment of creeping, it is not surprising that the infant will attempt to progress up stairs. This behavior begins shortly before the time the child has learned to walk (Gesell and Ilg, 1946) and a study of the cinema records of 12 infants by Ames (1937) indicates that the movement patterns used in ascending stairs at this time are almost identical to those used by the same infants in creeping on a level floor.

Soon after independent walking is established, the young child will attempt to ascend stairs in an upright position if supported by an older person and shortly thereafter will attempt ascent alone if there is a hand rail available to offer some support. The foot pattern used by young children just beginning to climb stairs differs from the alternating foot method used by adults in that the young novice will advance the same foot each time with the trailing foot brought up and placed on the riser beside the lead foot before the next step is taken. Thus the initial stair climbing pattern involves marking time on each step and is normally continued by most infants for several months until strength, balance, and coordination have developed to the extent that the adult alternate foot pattern can be negotiated successfully.

As with walking, a considerable variability exists among children as to the time at which they are able to climb stairs. With help, young children will usually ascend stairs in an upright position between 18 and 20 months of age. The problem of descent, however, is not mastered at the same rate as is ascent so that it is not unusual for a child to creep or walk up a short flight of stairs, if such is available, and then cry indignantly because he does not know how to get down. In general, descent, when it is first mastered, consists of crawling down the stairs backwards and, even when the child has achieved the skill to ascend stairs independently in the upright position, it is not unusual for him to make his descent by crawling down backwards.

A number of investigators have made independent observations of the development of stair climbing skill in youngsters and report similar types of activities used in the progressive development of the skill. After observing 98 children ranging in age from 26 to 74 months, Wellman (1937) noted that 50 percent of the children were successful at negotiating the various performance levels involved in stair climbing at certain ages. These she referred to as the "motor age" at which one might normally expect such a performance level. Her achievement levels and ages at which they were found to appear in 50 percent of her subjects are listed in Table 2. The youngsters were tested on their ability to negotiate both a short flight (3 steps) and a long flight (11 steps) of stairs.

Table 2
Stair Climbing Achievements of Preschool Children*

Stages in Ascending and Descending Steps	Motor Age in Months			
	Ascending		Descending	
	Short Fl.	Long Fl.	Short Fl.	Long Fl.
Mark time, without support	27	29	28	34
Alternate feet, with support	29	31	48	48
Alternate feet, without support	31	41	49	55

---

* From Béth L. Wellman, "Motor Achievements of Preschool Children." *Child. Educ.*, 13:311-316, 1937. Reprinted by permission of the Association for Childhood Education International, 3615 Wisconsin Avenue N.W., Washington, D.C.

The sequential stages listed by Wellman give evidence of successively more mature methods of negotiating stairs and are substantiated by the observations of Bayley (1935). However, the latter investigator noted that the children whom she observed tended to reach the various levels of achievement at a slightly earlier age. This finding is not out of line with the earlier reported differences in the ages in which the various progressive stages in walking were observed to occur in children in Minnesota (Shirley, 1931) and in California (Bayley, 1935). In this comparative instance, the California infants tended to achieve the skills necessary for both prone and upright locomotion at a slightly earlier age than those in Minnesota. These findings, in conjunction with the earlier achievements of stair climbing skills by the California children, would seem to indicate that there may be some regional differences in the onset of motor skills. Were comparative height and weight data available, it would also be interesting to analyze these data in terms of regional differences.

Considerable variability is reported to exist among studied children with respect to the age at which the various sequential stages are mastered by the children. Also there are considerable differences in the amount of time a child may utilize a certain technique as the primary means of negotiating stairs until the adult pattern is achieved (Wellman, 1937; Bayley, 1935). Moreover, there are inherent levels of difficulty in the length of the stairs to be negotiated and also in the height of the stair risers. Stairs with lower risers, so that they are more in proportion to the child's size, are mastered at an earlier age than stairs of adult size. Using an experimental staircase, Gesell and Thompson (1934) found that stair climbing behavior of the creeping type began in children between the ages of 40 to 50 weeks and, by 56 weeks of age, 53 percent of the infants were able to creep up a staircase constructed of four shorter risers. On the basis of these observations and the fact that studies tend to report averages based on group data, the standards of stair climbing performance established by various investigators should not be regarded as a rigid developmental schedule for the normal child but rather as a guide to the sequence and general time of appearance of such patterns in the motor development of children.

In general, studies of the development of ability in stair climbing indicate that: (1) ascending skill at a given level is achieved prior to descending abilities at the same level of achievement; (2) the child is able to accomplish an activity of a given level with help before he is able to perform the same activity alone; (3) at each level of achievement, the child will be able to negotiate a shorter flight of stairs before he is able to do so with a longer flight; and, (4) stairs with lower risers can be mastered, at each level of achievement, prior to those of adult height.

In ladder climbing, as in stair climbing, the developmental sequence involves leading with the same foot and marking time on each rung before the more mature technique of alternating feet is attempted with the skill of ascending a ladder being achieved before the youngster attempts to descend a ladder of equal length and rung placement. The distance between the rungs of the ladder seems to have a marked effect upon climbing performance and this is to be expected, since the normal distance separating the rungs of a ladder is greater than that of stair risers. Furthermore, a ladder may be placed at varying angles and the greater the inclination the greater the height and the greater the strength requirement in both the arms and legs to support and propel the body. An apparent association that seems to be made by all children is that of the height of the climb with the difficulty of ascent. Children who employed advanced climbing techniques when operating at low heights have been noted to revert to more cautious movements on all fours when the heights they are to climb are materially increased (Guttridge, 1939).

When general climbing ability is studied using such equipment as stairs, packing boxes, inclined planks, jungle gyms, and similar apparatus, a steady increase in climbing proficiency is noted between the ages of 3 to 6 years. Guttridge (1939) used such equipment to survey the climbing performance of approximately 2000 youngsters ranging in age from 2 to 7 years and found that by the time these children were 6 years old over 90 percent of them could be classified as reasonably proficient climbers. There were wide differences among the children in climbing ability at every age, with the boys being slightly superior to the girls at 2, 3, and 6 years while the sexes tended to be of equal ability at 4 and 5 years of age.

JUMPING AND HOPPING

The development of jumping and hopping involves fairly complicated modifications of the walking and running movement patterns. Since the jump necessitates elevation of the body off the ground for a longer period than is required for the run, greater strength is required to exert sufficient force and more complicated balancing adjustments are required both to maintain an acceptable body position while the body is in the air and to accommodate the body to the immediate deceleration of landing. Jumping occurs when the body is lifted completely off the ground by the action of one or both legs and the landing is made on one or both feet. Hopping, then, is a more complicated version of the jump for the body is lifted off the ground by the action of one foot and the landing is made on the same foot so that a higher degree of strength is required and a finer adjustment of balance is necessary to achieve a successful landing on the relatively small one-foot base. The leap is a specialized version of the run with the take-off being made from one foot and the landing on the alternate foot. However, the distance covered is so much greater in the leap than in any step of the run that the strength and balance requirements are closer to those of the jump.

a. Jumping. The first stage in jumping is considered to be the exaggerated step down from a higher level to a lower one so that the onset of jumping and descending stairs has the same origin and, of course, the same occurrence in time. When a momentary period occurs during which the child is not supported in his progress from a higher to a lower level a downward leap or a one-foot jump is executed (Figure 16). Here the child must have achieved enough strength and balance to accommodate the gravity-generated force of his descent to immediate deceleration on a narrow one-foot base.

At about the same time that the child is experimenting with one-foot jumps from heights with help, he has been independently jumping up and down on the floor with both feet used simultaneously. Although a two-foot landing is more stable, the two-foot take-off presents coordination problems that are new to the child since all his previous locomotion techniques have been based upon single, not simultaneous, limb propulsion. It is not surprising, therefore, that the one-foot take-off and landing is replaced by the one-foot take-off and two-foot landing. However, the young child must first develop enough strength to produce the necessary body elevation and speed of limb movement that is required for the one-foot take-off and two-foot landing. Clearly, also, a higher level of neuromuscular coordination is required for this latter type of jump. On the basis of its ontogenetic development, the most difficult type of jump for distance would appear to be the standing broad jump with its two-foot take-off and landing (Figure 17).

There would appear to be almost a parallel development in both stair climbing and jumping off heights, which may have its basis in the similar origin of the two activities or may just be a reflection of the expansion in the variety of activities with which the child is

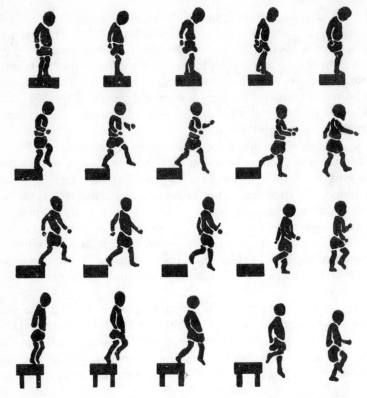

Figure 16.   Illustrations of the inability of the very young child (Willie) to jump from two feet simultaneously. **Rows 1 and 2,** stepping off an elevation at 17 months of age. **Row 3,** momentary suspension during a jump made at 18 months. **Row 4,** signs of incipient two-footed jumping at 21 months. Observe beginning shoulder girdle and arm retraction. (From F. A. Hellebrandt, G. L. Rarick, R. Glassow, and M. L. Carns, "Physiological Analysis of Basic Motor Skills. I. Growth and Development of Jumping." **Amer. J. Phys. Med.,** 40:14-25, 1961. By permission of the publisher, Williams and Wilkins.)

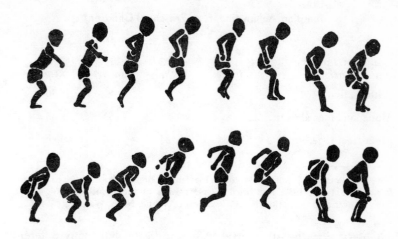

Figure 17.   **Row 1,** the earliest jump from a two-footed
               take-off observed in David at 32 months of
               age. **Row 2,** standing broad jump at the age
               of 3 years. Note the same shoulder girdle
               and arm retraction seen in Figure 16. (From
               F. A. Hellebrandt, G. L. Rarick, R. Glassow,
               and M. L. Carns, "Physiological Analysis of
               Basic Motor Skills. I. Growth and Develop-
               ment of Jumping." **Amer. J. Phys. Med.,**
               40:14-25, 1961. By permission of the pub-
               lisher, Williams and Wilkins.)

experimenting at this time. The "motor age" at which 50 percent
of the youngsters observed by Wellman (1937) were able to successfully perform the various achievement levels of jumping from
various heights is reproduced in Table 3. It may be noted that the
earliest efforts were executed with the modified step-down movement
and that the children were able to perform the activity at a given
height and level of achievement with help before they were able to
execute the skill alone. The more mature method of jumping with
two feet together did not appear until some time after successful
one-foot take-off had been achieved at the same height.

Table 3
Jumping Achievements of Preschool Children*

| | Motor Age in Months | | | |
Stages in Jumping (from heights)	8 inches	12 inches	18 inches	28 inches
With help			27	36
Alone, one foot ahead		27	31	43
Alone, feet together	33	34	37	46

* From Beth L. Wellman, "Motor Achievements of Preschool Children." *Child. Educ.*, 13:311-316, 1937. Reprinted by permission of the Association for Childhood Education International, 3615 Wisconsin Avenue, N.W., Washington, D.C.

Observations by other investigators indicate that many different types of jumps are being explored by the child at about the same time. Normal progress in the various types of jumps is illustrated in Figure 18. It may be noted that jumping over a barrier, in this instance a rope, appears to occur somewhat after jumps from height and jumps for distance have been mastered to a certain degree. Another investigator, Guttridge (1939), has observed that these types of jumps appear to be a complicated problem for youngsters and found it was not uncommon for 4-year-old children to have difficulty with jumping over barriers. This same study revealed that, in general, 42 percent of preschool children are able to jump well at 3 years of age while 72 percent may be considered to be skillful jumpers at 4½ years, with 80 percent of them having reasonably good mastery of jumping skills one-half year later.

The development of jumping has been summarized by Hellebrandt et al. (1961), with special emphasis on the standing broad jump, on the basis of the cinematographical records of 47 boys ranging in age from 14 months to 11 years. These investigators conclude that:

1. Jumping is a phylogenetic acquisition which unfolds progressively *pari passu* with growth and development of mechanisms capable of mobilizing the mechanical forces required.
2. Stepping off elevations precedes ability to jump by simultaneously extending both lower extremities.
3. Protection of the integrity of the weight-bearing limbs is insured

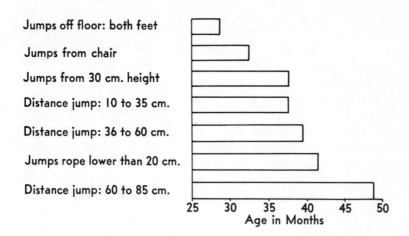

Figure 18.   Progress in various jumping skills. (Adapted
from data by Nancy Bayley, "The Develop-
ment of Motor Abilities in the First Three
Years." **Monogr. Soc. Res. Child Develpm.,**
1(1):1-26, 1935.)

from the onset of jumping by automatic alignment of the lower
extremities to receive the impact of landing most advantageously.
4. The upper extremities serve first as brakes by moving in a direction
opposite to the line of motion, then as coronal plane stabilizers,
and finally as augmenters of the momentum generated by the
extensor thrust of the legs.
5. The head moves spontaneously to maintain a normal relation to
gravity and in so doing probably evokes the tonic neck reflex and
labyrinthine reflexes and optical righting reflexes.
6. There is no suppression of sagittal plane head movement with
growth and development.
7. The learned aspects of skill cannot be differentiated unequi-
vocally from autonomous modulations in the patterning of neuromuscular response.*

---

* Excerpt from F. A. Hellebrandt, G. L. Rarick, R. Glasgow, and M. L. Carns,
"Physiological Analysis of Basic Motor Skills: 1. Growth and Development of
Jumping." *Amer. J. Phys. Med.*, 40:14-25, 1961. By permission of the publishers.

b. Hopping. As previously mentioned, hopping involves the elevation of the body from the ground by one foot and the successful landing on the same foot. One investigator considers the sequential development of hopping to involve a gradual transition from an early irregular series of jumps to a more coordinated, regular pattern and manner of movement (Guttridge, 1939), while another believes hopping on two feet, which occurs earlier than hopping on one foot, to be part of the sequential development of this skill (McCaskill and Wellman, 1938). It is obvious that the development of balance, as well as the necessary strength to elevate the mass of the body with one foot, is required before any skill may be achieved in hopping. Table 4 clearly indicates that hopping on both feet is mastered some time before the child is able to hop an equal distance using only one foot.

Table 4

Hopping Achievements of Preschool Children*

	Motor Age in Months	
Hopping, Steps	*Both Feet*	*One Foot*
1 to 3	38	43
4 to 6	40	46
7 to 9	41	55
10 or more	42	60

* From Beth L. Wellman, "Motor Achievements of Preschool Children." *Child. Educ.*, 13:311-316, 1937. Reprinted by permission of the Association for Childhood Education International, 3615 Wisconsin Avenue, N.W., Washington, D.C.

Static balance on one foot is, according to Bayley (1935), not achieved until the infant is approximately 29 months old and it is not until almost 21 months later, at approximately 50 months, that the average performer is able to hop up to 2 meters on the right foot. The intricacies of hopping, however, are not fully mastered at this time, for Breckenridge and Vincent (1949) point out that it is not until 6 years of age that most children can be considered to hop with skill and, even at this age, the range of skill varies from those extremely inept or refusing to make the effort to those children who are excellent performers. Once some skill has been mastered in hopping, the child tends to experiment with a large number of variations, such as hopping sidewise, backwards, and changing facing, and incorporates these into such games as hopscotch.

SKIPPING AND GALLOPING

The skills of skipping and galloping are built into the walking and running patterns by the additional introduction of modified jumping movements. Galloping combines the basic patterns of the walk and the leap while the skip consists of a hop interspaced in the walk pattern with the familiar "step-hop" of so many folk dances being a rhythmic variation of the skip pattern. The relatively late appearance of these skills in the motor behavior of the young child may be expected in view of the fact that they require the development of the balancing mechanisms at, or above, the level of hopping and that the movement sequences involved in their successful performance are new to the child even though their separate components have already been mastered.

Galloping is learned by most children by pounding to the strong beat of the music with the same foot or by periodically introducing a leaping step into their run. Gradually, the children will master the technique and degree of balance required to consistently throw their body weight onto the forward foot and then they begin to experiment with sidewise and backward variations in addition to the first learned forward progression. Guttridge's observations (1939) reveal the relatively late acquisition of this skill although it tends to appear slightly sooner than skipping. This investigator noted that 43 percent of the children at 4 years of age could be classified as having learned to gallop with the percentage increasing to 78 by 5 years although skillful galloping is not achieved by most children until they are approximately 6½ years of age.

A type of shuffle, which is performed by the child at approximately 38 months, may be considered to be a forerunner of the first skipping movements. More frequently, the early skipping movements are considered to be those which involve a skip on one foot while the other performs only a walking pattern. Such activity has been noted as occurring around 43 months with the full blown alternate foot pattern of skipping not being achieved until the child is approximately 60 months old (Wellman, 1937). Children, however, are not content with the mere acquisition of the basic alternate foot pattern of skipping but also explore variations involving changes of direction and tempo. The relatively complex nature of skipping is indicated by the fact that only 14 percent of 4-year-olds and 22 percent of 5-year-olds were considered by Guttridge (1939) as skipping well. By the time the observed children were 6 years old, 90 percent of them were classified as being able to skip but, even at this time, the variation in performance among the children was still very great.

KICKING

By the time the child is two years old, his balancing mechanisms have developed to the extent that he is able to maintain an upright position when balanced on one foot and still impart some degree of force to an object, such as a ball, with the other foot. During the early attempts, the range of action of the propulsive leg is very limited and the first kicks are executed with no backswing and very little follow through so that the object to be kicked must be directly in front of the foot or contact will not be made. Gradually as a higher degree of balance and strength are developed, the range of movement increases, first with a backswing originating from the knee, then the hip joint, and finally with a full leg backswing which includes a concomitant forward body lean by the time the child is 6 years (Deach, 1951).

As the range of the backswing increases and amount of force generated increases, the follow through must naturally also be augmented to absorb the generated forces and maintain balance. Therefore, from the early beginnings of a stationary upper torso with arms at the side, the arms become increasingly used for maintenance of balance, with marked arm-foot opposition being evident at the age of 6 years (Halverson and Roberton, 1966). Furthermore, the body increasingly tilts backwards during the follow through to compensate for the increasingly greater termination angle of the propulsive leg.

THROWING

In a sense, the beginnings of the throwing pattern may be considered to originate in the first releases of an object held by an infant. However, the skill of throwing effectively, namely, the ability to project an object accurately and with sufficient force through space, requires coordination of many distinct mechanisms which require many years of experimentation and practice on the part of the child before a mature pattern is developed. At approximately 6 months of age, many children are able to perform a crude and unrefined throw involving limited and isolated use of the throwing arm when the child is in a sitting position. In general, children are able to give a reasonably well defined direction to a thrown ball shortly before the first year. Further observation reveals that both distance and direction improve during the second year but that the throwing pattern tends to remain quite immature, consisting mainly of stiff, jerky movements of the arms with little or no effective use being made of foot or trunk movements (Gesell and Thompson, 1934).

Using a number of trained observers to rate the children included in her study, Guttridge (1939) noted that none of the children was rated as throwing well at 2 and 3 years of age. At 4 years, only 20 percent of the children were considered to be proficient in throwing while improvement tended to become more rapid after this time so that 74 percent were rated as proficient between the ages of 5 to 5½ years and the percentage increased to 84 by the sixth year. Wide variations in skill level among the children were observed at all ages with judgments ranging from very awkward to highly proficient even at 6 years when a relatively high level of skill had been attained.

A more objective measure of throwing ability is the distance the individual is able to throw objects of certain sizes. This type of testing procedure was used by Wellman (1937) to assess the "motor ages" at which 98 children were able to throw two balls, one of 9½ inch circumference and the other of 16¼ inch circumference. Her results are recorded in Table 5.

An exhaustive study was made by Wild (1938) of the development of throwing behavior in which the combinations of movement patterns of the arms and body were analyzed by means of cinemat-

Table 5
Ball Throwing Achievements of Preschool Children*

Distance of throw, feet	Motor Age in Months	
	Small ball (9½ in.)	Large ball (16¼ in.)
4 to 5	30	30
6 to 7	33	43
8 to 9	44	53
10 to 11	52	63
12 to 13	57	above 72
14 to 15	65	
16 to 17	above 72	

* From Beth L. Wellman, "Motor Achievements of Preschool Children." *Child. Educ.*, 13:311-316, 1937. Reprinted by permission of the Association for Childhood Education International, 3615 Wisconsin Avenue, N.W., Washington, D.C.

ographic records taken of children during the performance of a throw. Although the study was of the cross-sectional type, the children at each age level were carefully selected on the basis of the achievement of normal physical, motor, mental, and personality development at the time of the study. This selection involved a total of 32 children comprising a boy and a girl at each 6-month-age level within the age range of 2 to 7 years. Each subject was asked to perform three overhand throws which were filmed and subsequently carefully analyzed.

Analysis of the data revealed four distinct types of throws which appeared to be closely associated with particular age groups. The least mature type of throw predominates at the ages of 2 and 3 and involves movements of the arm and body which are confined mainly to the anterioposterior plane. In starting the first phase of this throwing pattern, the arm is drawn up either frontally or obliquely with a corresponding extension of the trunk until the object to be thrown is at a point high above the shoulders. With the delivery, the trunk straightens with a forward carry of the shoulders as the arm comes through fairly stiffly in a downward motion. During the entire throw, both feet remain firmly in place and the body facing toward the direction of the throw is also maintained.

The second pattern of throw was typical of the $3\frac{1}{2}$ to 5 year age range and was distinguished from the first type of throw by the execution of both the arm and the body movements in a horizontal plane rather than the previously used anterioposterior plane. Although the feet continue to remain together and in place during the entire throw, rotation of the body is first to the right in preparing to throw and then to the left as the ball is delivered with the right hand. The arm action is slightly flatter than the previous arm pattern but greater in force attained from the forward and downward follow through.

The most conspicuous change in pattern during the fifth and sixth years involves the introduction of a step forward with the right foot as the ball is delivered with the right hand. This marks the third stage. In the preparatory phase of the throw, the weight is retained on the left, or rear, foot while the body is rotated to the right and the arm is brought obliquely upward and over the shoulder so that it is in a flexed and retracted position. During delivery, the child steps forward on the right foot while the body rotates to the left and the arm swings forward in either an oblique or lateral movement about the shoulder joint. Upon completion of the throw, the body facing is partially to the left in contrast to the earlier forward facing in the preceding throwing patterns.

The mature throwing pattern is the fourth in the sequence identified by Wild and was used by all the boys in this study of $6\frac{1}{2}$ years and older. Again the main change from the preceding pattern is in the use of the base of support to provide opposition of movement so that greater power can be obtained from the throw. In this instance, the weight is transferred to the right foot during the preparatory phase and the left foot moves forward and receives the weight during the delivery phase of the throw. Such action enables a marked trunk rotation to occur and this, coupled with the horizontal adduction of the arm during the forward swing, enables the child to achieve the maximal use of body leverage for attaining speed at the most distal segment, in this instance, the hand. Although the boys achieved the adult pattern of overhand throw, the girls in Wild's study did not progress beyond the third stage in either arm or foot action or both. It is not uncommon for even adult women never to achieve the mature overhand throw pattern although it is usually found in skilled females.

In general, Wild (1938) concluded that there were two main developmental trends in the sequential movement patterns of throwing: namely, (1) the gradual shift of movements from a predominantly anterioposterior plane to a horizontal plane; and (2) the transition from the use of an unchanging base of support to a shifting base on the same side as the throwing arm followed by the transference of weight in a much more stable and functional arm-foot opposition relationship. Wild further noted that each of the successive throwing patterns exhibited a more effective means of mechanical projection on the basis of marked increase in the ability to develop acceleration in the ball.

CATCHING

The child has become very proficient in reaching for and grasping stationary objects by the time he is 2 years old but moving objects require adjustments for, and some understanding of, time-space relationships before any proficiency is achieved in catching them. Attempts at stopping a rolling ball or other moving objects can be considered to be initial attempts at catching. Perhaps the most successful of these early attempts at catching occurs when a ball is rolled toward the child as it is seated on the floor with legs spread apart. The ball may then be stopped by the hands or corralled by the legs fairly readily. With sufficient practice the child will gradually be able to synchronize the movements of the arms with the speed of the ball and the hands can then reach around the ball and stop it.

A ball tossed into the air is influenced by the effects of gravity so that catching an aerial ball presents a more complicated task than the relatively simpler adjustment to variations in speed and direction in the horizontal plane such as is characteristic of a rolling ball. The first attempts at catching an aerial ball usually consist of simply holding the arms stiffly out-stretched in front of the body. Little or no effort is made to move the body to adjust to the flight of the ball and, even when the toss lands directly on the arms, their stiffness or delayed shovelling action usually results in failure to retain possession of the ball. Gradually the child begins to develop a sense of timing and the arms are relaxed slightly so that tosses directly into the arms are scooped up against the body with the arms and hands working as a unit. Very gradually, also, the child begins to be able to judge and adjust to increasingly greater deviations in the position of the aerial ball and will move his body to try to get into the most favorable catching position.

With increasing age, the catching pattern changes to one in which the elbows are still kept in front of the body but the hands are positioned in opposition to one another in a similar manner to the position of the jaws in a vise. Gradually this pattern gives way to the mature form where the elbows are to the sides of the body and the hands are cupped with either the thumbs or little fingers together, depending upon the position of the ball, to receive the ball. The arms at the sides position allows for a greater degree of "give" in arm movement in absorbing the force of the ball. As with throwing, some girls never acquire the mature two-handed catching pattern and tend to use the vise positioning of the hands to catch the ball, although the predominating trend involves arms at the side of the body. Depending upon the size of the object, variations such as one-handed catching are attempted as soon as some confidence is achieved in judgment of speed and direction.

Table 6

Ball Catching Achievements of Preschool Children*

	Motor Age in Months	
Method of catching the ball (success in 2 or 3 trials)	*Large ball* (16¼ in.)	*Small ball* (9½ in.)
Arms straight	34	37
Elbows in front of body	44	50
Elbows at side of body	68	—

* From Beth L. Wellman, "Motor Achievements of Preschool Children." *Child. Educ.*, 13:311-316, 1937. Reprinted by permission of the Association for Childhood Education International, 3615 Wisconsin Avenue, N.W., Washington, D.C.

The relatively slow acquisition of catching skills is illustrated by the findings of a study by Wellman (1937) with the same sized small and large balls that were used for throwing (Table 6). As may be expected, skill is attained at a certain level of performance with the large ball before the same level is achieved with the small ball. In general, proficiency in catching is achieved by only 29 percent of 4-year-olds, 56 percent of 5-year-olds, while at 6 years the proportion has increased to only 63 percent (Guttridge, 1939).

BALL BOUNCING

Ball bouncing has its origins in the casual or deliberate dropping of the ball to cause it to bounce. From this simple, single bounce a very gradual improvement occurs in the number of times a child is able to tap the ball until control is lost or the taps no longer impart enough force to the ball for it to bounce to any reasonable height. The mature, multiple, controlled bounce requires that the proportionate size of the hand and ball are such that some control over direction is forthcoming in the placement of the hand in relation to the center of mass of the ball. Furthermore, the hand should meet the ball on the upward portion of the bounce for a maximum contact period rather than "chase" the ball when on its downward path as is typical of the unskilled performer.

Although the two hand bounce would seem to offer advantages in that a bigger hand surface is available for contact, and hence control, of the ball and more force could also be applied to the ball, it is in fact inferior to the one hand bounce in that the use of two hands restricts the positioning of the ball in relationship to the body to a position directly in front of the body. Furthermore, the time of contact and the amount of force exerted by each hand must be extremely concise and well synchronized for the achievement of any degree of control over the direction of the ball. Therefore, it is not surprising that the one hand multiple bounce is mastered by children prior to a two hand bounce.

However, the size of the ball in relation to the size of the hand is an important consideration in the development of ball bouncing. Children are able to bounce a small ball of 9½ inch circumference for a distance of one to three feet at approximately 27 months of age using one hand. The distance is increased to four to five feet by the age of 40 months and it is not until 46 months of age that the child is able to bounce a larger ball of 16¼ inch circumference over an equal distance using the two hand bounce. The larger ball, however, presents problems of control and sufficient strength to the young child, for it is not until approximately 71 months of age, or 45 months after bouncing a small ball for a distance of one to three feet, that the child is able to bounce the large ball a distance of one to three feet using one hand (Wellman, 1937).

STRIKING

Striking develops from a throw action in the anterioposterior plane and is generally associated with anger or resentment on the part of the infant. It is not unusual to see angry children throw "nothing" at each other or even at an adult. Gradually such action is restricted to situations in which contact can be achieved with an object but the type of contact has the texture of a push rather than an actual hit. The overhand arm action is still used at the time actual hitting with one hand occurs but is gradually replaced by an underarm, or sidearm, striking action. The position of the object does, however, still influence the angle of approach of the arm. The addition of the other patterns augments the range of approach.

A study by Halverson and Roberton (1966) shows that a directional goal such as "Can you hit the ball to your dad?" elicits a sidearm striking pattern with a light plastic paddle when a tennis ball is suspended at waist high level at the age of 3 years. Furthermore, at this same age, children can successfully contact a softly tossed aerial ball with a one hand sidearm swing but experience difficulty in contact using a two handed sidearm swing for, although the pattern is well defined, the swing is initiated too early. In general, well defined sidearm striking patterns are used by children beginning at approximately 3 years of age as long as successful contact is achieved but substitution of a less mature form of pattern or of another pattern is almost immediately made when failure re-

sults under stress, the problem is beyond the ability of the youngster, or the equipment is too long or heavy. Children of this age
also appear to experience less difficulty in contacting a ball tossed
with an underhand pattern than one with an overarm pattern even
when the velocity of the toss is as constant as possible. This type of
experience is limited for children of this age since the cooperation
of an adult is required. It assumes importance in the peer group
when the child becomes of school age.

SWIMMING

One of the earliest ages at which training in swimming has been
attempted was undertaken by McGraw (1935) in her experiments
with Johnny and Jimmy, the former being the twin receiving training while the latter received no training. Instruction in swimming
for Johnny was begun when he was 231 days, or approximately 8
months old, with the aid of a strap support to prevent his complete
submersion so that he was able to hold his head out of the water.
However, lowering the supporting strap so that greater use could
be made of the arms revealed that Johnny preferred to swim
with his face under the water. Therefore, at the age of 290 days, or
around $9\frac{1}{2}$ months, Johnny was submerged without artificial support and by the time he was 17 months old was able to swim from
12 to 15 feet, which was the distance permitted by one breath.

Observations of primitive children who are allowed to play in
the water from early infancy indicate that there are few, if any,
who are not able to swim well at 5 years (Mead, 1930). Some recent
work with preschool children indicates that it is not unusual for
3-year-olds to develop reasonably good swimming skills and it is
possible that there may be real advantages with regard to physique
for the introduction of swimming at this time. Rarick (1954) points
out that the remaining baby fat would tend to add to the bouyancy
of these younger children and the short legs would reduce drag.
Furthermore, the early introduction of swimming would preclude,
or offer less opportunity for, the development of negative attitudes
to water which become more dominant as the child becomes older.
However, when observed in situations without formal instruction,

children under five years of age seem to prefer to splash and play in the water with little concern for learning to swim, whereas after this age interest in learning to swim increases greatly as does the rate of progress in learning to swim.

OTHER ACTIVITIES

Once the child has learned to walk most of his physical activities during the next four years are concerned with play, to the extent that investigators in the field of child development consider play to be the most important business of childhood. Toys are, at one and the same time, the instruments of play and the tools by which children develop their gross and fine motor abilities. Kawin (1934) has classified toys on the basis of five types of play situations in which they can be used and suggests that an adequate selection of each type of toy is vital to the development of the child in each of the five areas. Selections should, therefore, include: (1) toys for developing bodily strength and growth in a variety of physical skills; (2) creative constructive toys, such as blocks, clay, hammers, nails, and saws; (3) toys for dramatization and imitation, such as miniature houses, automobiles, stores, forts, and farms; (4) toys emphasizing the artistic, such as toy musical and rhythmic instruments, and art and handicraft materials; and (5) toys for promoting intellectual development which might include animal or bird games, anagrams, map puzzles, and travel games.

Children tend to respond to different play materials in a different manner at various age levels. Between the ages of 2 to 6 years the most frequently used indoor play materials are, according to Van Alystne (1932), blocks, clay, and doll-corner materials. Furthermore, children tend to use the same materials in different ways with advancing years, indicating a continuity of preference for favorite toys which points to a recommendation of a smaller number of well-selected, durable toys in preference to a large number of limited-use, easily broken toys. From the previous discussion of throwing, catching, bouncing, kicking, and striking, it is quite obvious that balls are also a favorite toy of children of this age and have many uses as well as being reasonably durable.

Wheel toys are very popular and extensively used by children when available. These include the push and pull type of toy, the kiddie car, wagon, tricycle, roller skates, and bicycle. Recently a large number of the push and pull type of toys have become battery operated, which, although they may create an incentive for the child to chase the toy, do remove a great deal of the opportunity for using the back and leg muscles for propulsive power as well as reducing the exploratory learnings of the child into the manner in which such propulsive force has to be applied. Fortunately the larger wheel toys still allow such developmental opportunities until late childhood when the mechanized go-cart again is a temptation.

An extensive investigation of the developmental sequences which occur during the process of learning to operate a wagon has been made by Jones (1939). He noted that children of 21 to 26 months will manipulate the parts of the wagon and push it back and forth repeatedly in an unskilled manner. The next two months may see the child getting into the wagon in the typical propulsive position with one knee on the wagon bed and the other on the ground but no effort is made to propel the wagon. Subsequent to this period and until the thirty-sixth month, practicing of the propelling skill is undertaken in the typical propulsion position. There is a gradual unification of the skills involved into an increasingly skillful pattern so that by the time the child is 4 years old the specific skills of propelling and manipulating a wagon are well established and the child is able to operate in terms of ideas he wishes to effect rather than simply concentrating on the motor act involved in the operation of the wagon.

Similar behavioral changes have been observed in children learning to ride tricycles. If children have been exposed to wheel toys from an early age, it is not surprising to find them showing a marked facility in their operation, and under these circumstances, 2-year-old youngsters may exhibit considerable skill in handling tricycles, being able to steer, back, and manage sharp turns with speed and accuracy. In general, most children can ride a tricycle proficiently at 3 years of age and it is not infrequent for youngsters of this age to have some ability in the management of two-wheeled scooters while reasonable skill in the operation of foot-operated automobiles is achieved by the age of 4 years. Bicycle riding is usually an achievement of later childhood when the·child is more capable of handling the vehicle in traffic. Children of 5 and 6 can ride small bicycles, however, if they have the opportunity to do so.

Although Johnny was trained by McGraw (1935) to roller skate at 2 years, it is more usual for children of 5 and 6 years to attain some proficiency in roller skating if they are given adequate opportunity to practice. Similarly, in cold climates, ice skating is an activity in which some degree of mastery is possible at this age level and bob sleds, toboggans, and skis replace wagons and tricycles in the snowy, winter months.

BALANCE

As with the acquisition of walking, running, and jumping and the numerous locomotor variations of these skills, the problem of balance is vitally important in the acquiring of skill in roller skating, ice skating, skiing, and operating two-wheeled vehicles. The development of balance itself has been the subject of numerous studies. However, the complexity of balance and the wide range of ability from one age level to another has resulted in very low inter-

Table 7

Dynamic Balance on a Walking Board*

	Age in Months
Tries to stand on walking board	22.5
Walking with one foot on board	27.6
Standing on board with both feet	31.0
Attempts to step	32.8
Alternates feet part way	38.0
Alternates feet full length	56.0
Length in 6 to 9 secs.	59.5
Length in 3 to 5 secs.	66.0
Length in less than 3 secs.	80.0

* From Nancy Bayley, "A Scale of Motor Development." Institute of Child Welfare, University of California, Berkeley. By permission.

correlations of the various measures so that no single measure of balance can be considered to be useful for testing over a wide age range.

The walking board has, however, been used as a dynamic test of balance over a wider age range than any other measure but even here the size of the board, the manner of scoring, and the general procedure differ to such an extent that comparison of results obtained by different investigators is not feasible. In general, developmental sequence of dynamic balance and the age placement of the various levels obtained by Bayley using a walking board 2.5 meter long, 6 cm. wide, and 10 cm. high are typical of those obtained by other investigators (Table 7).

GENERAL MOTOR DEVELOPMENT

The tendency for certain phases in the developmental sequence to be achieved by children at approximately the same time has led a number of investigators to develop motor scales of performance indicating normative behavior in a wide variety of activities. The California Infant Scale of Motor Development, published in 1936 and based upon a somewhat select group of approximately 50 children, is indicative of this type of scale, which attempts to assess a general motor development rather than separate the various skills as has been done in the foregoing discussion (Table 8).

Although no distinction is generally made in the motor performance of boys and girls in most activities during infancy and early childhood because the differences are not very great, there are some events in which one sex tends to exceed the performance of the other in either maturity of pattern development or in objective measure. In the case of reports involving pattern development or subjective rating of skill level, there will, in the very nature of such procedures, be a substantial variability in the criteria of judgment so that this type of study will more frequently report sex differences. In one such investigation of skill levels girls are reported as tending to excel in hopping, skipping, and galloping while boys are superior in jumping and throwing from the ages of 2 to 7 years (Guttridge, 1939). A cinematographic study of children, aged 2 through 6 years, of the performance of throwing, catching, kicking, striking, and ball bouncing indicated that the boys were

Table 8

California Infant Scale of Motor Development*

Months	
16.5	Walks sideways
16.9	Walks backwards—several steps
20.3	Walks upstairs with help
24.3	Walks upstairs alone—marks time
28.0	Jumps off floor—both feet
29.2	Stands on one foot alone
30.1	Walks on tiptoe
32.1	Jumps from chair—26 cm. high
35.5	Walks upstairs—alternating forward foot
37.3	Distance jump—10 to 35 cm.
49.3	Hop on one foot—2 or 3 hops

* Excerpts from Nancy Bayley, *The California Infant Scale of Motor Development*. Berkeley: University of California Press, 1936. By permission of the publisher.

about one year in advance of the girls in pattern development and showed greater ability to move with an integrated body pattern in all activities except the multiple ball bounce (Deach, 1951). Objective measurements, however, generally reveal little difference between the sexes except in the throw for distance.

In general, the development of motor skills proceeds according to the laws which govern the physiological maturation of the child, with the development of movement patterns progressing from simple arm or leg actions to highly integrated total body coordinations. This increase in complexity of patterns of performance is defined by most investigators of sequential motor patterning in terms of stages of development, and seems to be more interrelated with physiological maturation than with chronological age. The extent of such relationships is highly debatable, however, on the basis of present knowledge, since physiological maturation does have substantial relationship with chronological age and the sequential patterning of motor behavior has also been associated with chronological age. Most of the information dealing with such development has been collected in cross-sectional studies whose main objective was to set up norms for various performance levels. With the availability of more refined cinematographic techniques and other recording devices such as electromyograms and electroencephalograms, the area of the relationship between physiological maturation and motor behavior patterning would seem to be an experimentally fruitful one, especially in terms of longitudinal studies.

CHAPTER VIII

MOTOR BEHAVIOR IN LATER CHILDHOOD

The relatively slow and constant growth trend of later childhood, extending approximately from 6 to 10 or 12 years of age, is terminated by the pubescent growth spurt. Although these years are ones of slow developmental change, it is a time of rapid learning (Goodenough, 1945) and what may be thought of as growth consolidation, characterized more by the perfection and stabilization of previously acquired skills and abilities rather that the emergence of new ones.

It is also the period in which the child moves from the sheltered home environment to the involved social climate of the school. Major adjustments are required to cope with the three outward thrusts that are the developmental tasks of this period, namely (1) the thrust from the home into the peer group; (2) the thrust into the realm of work and games, each of which requires added development of neuromuscular skills; and (3) the thrust into the world of adult concepts, which requires the gradual acquisition of the skills and art of logic, symbolism, and communication (Havighurst, 1950).

CHANGES IN SIZE AND BODY PROPORTIONS

The relatively slow and constant growth of this period is an important factor in improved motor functioning and coordination. Body size and proportions change gradually and so a nearly constant relationship is maintained in bone and tissue development. Therefore, the energies of growth can be directed toward perfecting the basic movement patterns that have been established during the period of early childhood and adapting and modifying them to meet an increasing variety of situations.

The limbs continue to grow proportionately more than the trunk

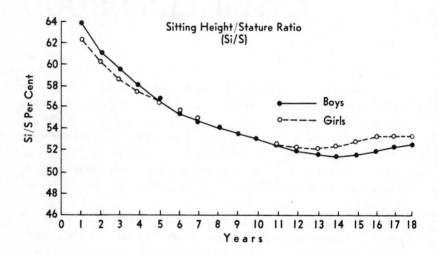

Figure 19.   The ratio of sitting height to stature at ages 1 to 18 inclusive. As the legs grow relatively longer, the ratio falls, rising again after puberty. (From Leona M. Bayer and Nancy Bayley, **Growth Diagnosis.** Chicago: The University of Chicago Press, 1959. By permission of the publisher.)

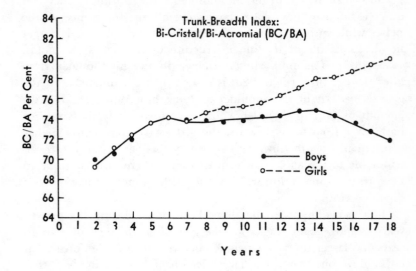

Figure 20.   The ratio of bi-cristal diameter to bi-acromial
diameter at ages 1 to 18 inclusive. As boys'
shoulders grow relatively wider, their ratio
falls. As girls' hips grow relatively broader,
the BC/BA curve for girls rises. (From Leona
M. Bayer and Nancy Bayley, **Growth Diagnosis.** Chicago: The University of Chicago
Press, 1959. By permission of the publisher.)

and this is particularly so for boys so that the relatively longer leg
length of the girls during infancy and early childhood tends to
disappear in later childhood. Thereafter, the boys exhibit comparatively greater leg length. This growth pattern is illustrated
by the ratio of sitting height to stature shown in Figure 19. Here
the decline in the ratio indicates that the legs are growing longer
relative to the sitting height up until the age of 11 years for the
girls and 14 for the boys. The subsequent slight rise in the ratio
for both sexes after these times marks the increase in trunk length
which occurs toward the end of the adolescent growth spurt.

Another sex difference that becomes more noticeable after the age of 6 years is that of the hip-shoulder ratio. During infancy and early childhood, boys have larger overall measurements of the pelvis while girls tend to be either relatively or absolutely larger in measurements of the inner structure of the pelvis (Reynolds, 1945, 1947). The proportional change in the hip-shoulder ratio after the age of 6 (Figure 20) is caused by a sex difference in the growth pattern of the shoulder and the hip. While the relative amount of gain in shoulder width is approximately the same for both sexes from 6 to 10 years, the girls make consistently higher gains in hip width during this time. Subsequent changes are attributable to the adolescent growth spurt, where girls continue to have greater gains in hip width while the boys increase markedly in shoulder width.

Other sex differences that have been noted during the growth years include larger thighs for the girls from the ages of 3 to 18 years and larger thoracic circumference and girth of the forearm in boys (Boynton, 1936). The larger length of forearm for boys that becomes noticeable during early childhood is maintained through adulthood. However, the sex differences that have been cited are slight in late childhood and there is little difference with respect to physique between boys and girls until preadolescent changes are manifested.

INDICES OF GROWTH AND MATURATION

The most commonly used indices for assessing the developmental age or physiological maturity of a growing child are: skeletal age, dental age, secondary sex character age, and morphological age. Skeletal age is the most generally used indicator of physiological maturity, since its effective range extends from birth through 18 years of age. Roentgenograms of the hand and wrist are the most commonly used technique for assessing the amount of ossification and the amount of ephiphyseal fusion, with skeletal maturity being achieved upon the completion of both processes. Figure 21 clearly illustrates that girls are more skeletally mature than boys from birth and they maintain this status to achieve maturity approximately 2 years earlier than boys.

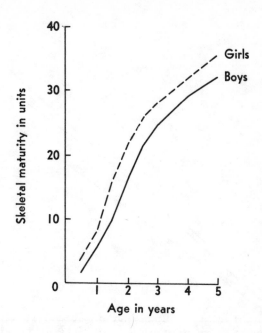

On the average, skeletal age and chronological age coincide but
any one individual may be normal, advanced, or retarded in skeletal age with respect to chronological age. There may also be fluctuations in the rate of skeletal maturing such as those illustrated in
Figure 22.

Dental age uses a principle similar to that of skeletal age and
employs the eruption or non-eruption of each tooth as the measure
of maturity. It has been found that the pattern of appearance of

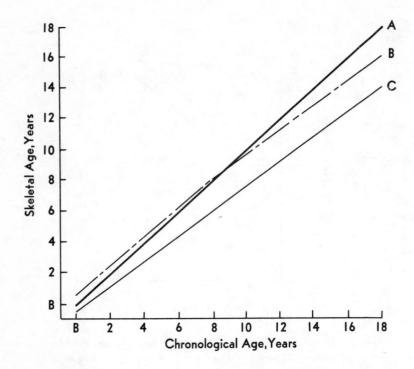

Figure 22.   Skeletal age plotted against chronological
age for 3 hypothetical persons. A, average of
standardising group throughout all growth
period; B, initially skeletally mature above
average, but passing later to below average;
C, consistently below average maturity (a
late maturer). (From J. M. Tanner, **Growth at
Adolescence.** Oxford, Eng.: Blackwell Scientific Publications, 1955. By permission of the
publisher.)

the two sets of teeth vary for the sexes. Although girls are more
mature than boys as measured by skeletal ossification and by permanent teeth eruption, boys are in advance of girls in the eruption

of the first, or deciduous, teeth from the first tooth to the last (Meredith, 1946). Using the data completed on 64 Fels Study children, Robinow et al. (1942) found that there were no differences between deciduous teeth eruption on the right and left sides but the upper-lower eruption differed with respect to the central incisors (lower first) and lateral incisors (upper first).

The eruption of the permanent teeth show marked sex differences, with every tooth appearing earlier, on the average, in girls than in boys. Furthermore, the timing of these differences ranges from 2 months for the first molars to 11 months for the canines (Hurme, 1949). Since the eruption of the deciduous teeth covers only the period from 6 months to 2 years and that of the permanent teeth from 6 to 13 years, dental age has not been used extensively for gauging maturity.

Secondary sex character age is based upon ratings for the stages of maturation of genital, pubic hair, and breast development and, as such, is applicable only to the periods of preadolescence and adolescence. Although the determination of secondary sex character age requires reasonably complicated procedures, this method of assessment of development has been frequently used and will be discussed more fully in dealing with the period of adolescence.

Morphological age employs height, weight, and various other anthropometric measures or combinations of these in relation to norms based upon chronologial age. The charts of growth in height, weight, and the common height-weight tables for the prediction of normal weight, are examples of this technique of assessing development. These types of measurements are the most easily obtained and the most obvious indicators of individual variations.

It may be well at this time to point out certain limitations that exist in the various measures of maturation. Available norms in all areas are based on cross-sectional studies of relatively homogeneous populations. All physical growth patterns, including those of the timing and sequence of ossification of the skeleton (Reynolds, 1943) and the eruption of teeth (Tisserand-Perrier, 1953) are to some degree hereditary in character. Thus norms for dental age especially, which are based on a relatively small sample, may be biased. Studies of various racial groups confirm the fact that human development follows a common pattern. Racial differences do exist, however, in actual size, proportions, and possibly timing. Norms are appropriate, therefore, only for populations comparable to those on which they were developed. One other limitation should be noted. Cross-sectionally developed norms all show straight-line growth whereas longitudinal studies demonstrate clearly that individual growth shows cycles of rapid and slow progress.

BODY BUILD

Closely allied to measures of morphological age is the body build of the child as it is based upon the interrelationships of height, weight, and various anthropometric measurements. Bayley and Davis (1935) found that the index of weight/length^2 was the most valid measure of lateral-linear tendencies in the body build during the first three years of life but that the indices obtained at these early ages were not predictive of what an individual's body build would be later in life. Figure 23 clearly indicates these changes in the growth pattern based upon the weight/length^2 ratios, of three girls who were taller than average. Here, as Bayley and Davis also found, chubbiness reached its peak between 9 and 12 months of age. Furthermore, although the curves do not cross from 28 weeks to 9 years, G43 was more chubby at 28 weeks than G44 at 5 years and G44 was decidedly more chubby at 28 weeks than G47 at 5 years. With regard to general body build, G43 was underweight for her height and age and had proportionately longer legs; G44 was of approximately normal proportions; while G47 was overweight for her height and age and had a comparatively large pelvis for her body length (Thompson, 1954).

Although weight increase is a correlate of growth, it is not necessarily indicative of growth since weight changes may be merely the result of changes in water content or of fatty deposits, both of which may be transitory modifications (Simmons and Todd, 1938). Weight has been found to be more variable and more indicative of nutritional status than any other physical measurement. In spite of the fact that the optimum weight of an individual depends upon the age, body build, and stature of an individual as well as on his nutrition, age norms for weight alone have been used as indicators

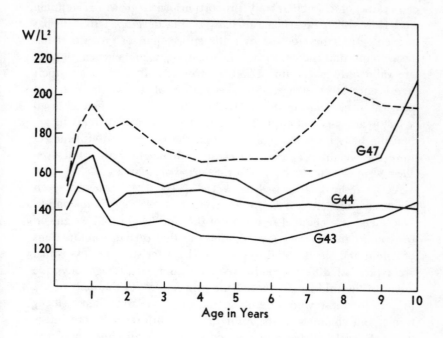

Figure 23.   Individual changes in weight: length² index with age. Girls G43, G44 and G47 are taller than average but of different body build. G43 is underweight for age and height; legs proportionately long. G44 approximates normal proportions. G47 is overweight for height; pelvis wide for body length. Dotted line represents index changes for short stocky girl. (From Helen Thompson, "Physical Growth." In L. Carmichael (Ed.), **Manual of Child Psychology.** New York: John Wiley & Sons, Inc., 1954. By permission of the publisher.)

of a child's development and nutritional status, particularly during the period of infancy.

Because of changing body proportions with growth (Hejinian and Hatt, 1929) no scheme of body typing developed to date has proven satisfactory for use over the entire span of growth. It has been found that indices such as stem length/recumbent length ratio are valid only at certain periods of growth and tend to lose their significance at other ages. An investigation of the whole period of physical growth was made by McCloy (1936) in which he employed a factor analysis technique to isolate the most useful items in appraising body type. He concluded that the two most useful indices were the weight$^{1/3}$/height and chest girth/height ratios, but even these were satisfactory only after the period of infancy.

A grid technique devised by Wetzel (1941, 1943) provides seven different growth channels for individuals of varying body builds. Placement in a channel results from plotting height and weight on the coordinates. Wetzel (1941) points out that certain combinations of height and weight tend to produce characteristic contours which are typical of different body types. Children of average physique fall into the middle channel of the grid while the channels to the left are for those who were obese and of progressively more stocky frame, and channels to the right for thin children of more linear frame. Wetzel believes that the body build for all children placed in the same channel on the basis of height and weight is essentially the same irrespective of their level of development. Furthermore, once a child's channel can be established at about 6 or 7 years, healthy children should be expected to maintain growth close to the limits imposed by the channel and thus to show consistent body build.

Since growth failure in the Wetzel technique is assessed from height and weight alone it is subject to marked limitations (Thompson, 1954). A more satisfactory technique developed by Pryor and Stolz (1933) used age, sex, height, and bi-iliac width for the prediction of optimum weight of children 6 to 16 years of age. No specific body typing results from the latter method, however.

A more comprehensive approach to body typing was undertaken by Sheldon and co-workers (1940), based upon adult male somatic characteristics, and using three main components and four second-order variables. These investigators relate the three components to the embryonic tissues, namely: the ectoderm, the mesoderm, and the endoderm. Ectomorphy is considered as characteristic of the body-type dominated by the central nervous system as shown by a linear, fragile body with a relatively large surface area; mesomorphy is characteristic of the bone, muscle, and connective tissue dominated body such as is shown by a heavy, hard, and rectangularly outlined body; and endomorphy is regarded as characteristic of the viscerally dominated body as evidenced by soft, rounded body regions. Within these three main components, the second-order variables are texture, or coarseness or fineness of the structure; dysplasia, or disharmony between the various parts of the body; hirsutism, or amount of body hair; and gynandromorphy, or degree of bisexuality. All these traits, both components and second-order variables, are rated on a seven point scale by anthroscopic and anthropometric methods. Adaptations of this body typing scheme have been made for women and children but to date these have not been widely used.

Sheldon himself somatotyped the boys and girls of the Oakland Growth Study. His final typing represented a composite for each individual developed from the serial photographs taken throughout the study as he considered this would better represent the genotype. A grouping of boys and of girls who were consistently superior or the reverse in motor abilities was made from these same subjects (Espenschade, 1940). Somatotypes of these latter individuals are summarized in Table 9. The superior performers among boys are high in mesomorphy and low in ectomorphy in comparison with the poor performers. Differences are less marked for girls as both groups are below average in mesomorphy. The poor performers are decidedly more endomorphic, however.

Table 9

Mean Sheldon Somatotype Ratings of Adolescent Boys and Girls High and Low in Physical Performances

	High			Low		
Boys	3.0	5.2	3.1	4.6	4.5	2.9
Girls	4.9	3.7	2.7	5.6	3.0	2.8

Still another approach to rating has been that of Bayley and Bayer (1946) who devised a five-area classification by which young adults may be evaluated according to the sex-appropriateness of their builds. The profile rating for androgynic patterns of body form developed by these investigators involves 14 items of measurement from photographic records which serve to categorize the individual into the five areas of hypermasculinity, masculinity, intermediate or bisexual, femininity, and hyperfemininity. Although the body typing of Sheldon has been related to motor performance, no study has yet been made relating Bayley and Bayer's rating to this area.

GROWTH AND MATURATION INDICES AND MOTOR PERFORMANCE

A relationship between body size and level of motor performance has long been recognized by individuals interested in physical abilities and one of the first systems of classifying children into homogeneous groups for games and athletic activities involved the use of chronological age, school grade, height, and weight (Reilly, 1917). The two most commonly used methods of classifying children and youth were developed independently by McCloy (1945) and by Neilson and Cozens (1934) with both using the factors of age, weight, and height. Each subjected records of thousands of children to statistical analysis and obtained multiple correlations ranging from .40 to .67 between various events and age, height, and weight. The classification formulas developed by these investigators were very similar, as follows:

McCloy: Classification Index $I = 20$ (Age)$+6$ (Height)$+$Weight
Neilson and Cozens: Revised Formula $= 20$ (Age)$+5.5$ (Height)$+$
1.1 (Weight).

Subsequently, these investigators modified their formulae for special age or sex groupings. McCloy (1945) concluded, for example, that height of elementary school boys added little to the prediction formula. He suggests that increases in body weight would normally reflect increases in the amount of muscle tissue if its proportion of approximately 40 percent of the body weight is retained. Furthermore, this increase in muscle tissue coupled with increased lever length resulting from growth in height should result in greater power and thus in higher motor achievement. Growth in height in the elementary school years is apparently reflected adequately by increase in weight so that the latter alone, with age, is predictive of performance.

In all of these earlier studies designed primarily to develop classification for physical activities, a wide range of performance measures were used and various age ranges were included. More recent studies, where computer analysis has been possible, have given more precise results. The importance of weight as an indicator of strength has been reaffirmed by Clarke and Carter (1959) who found, after experimenting with chronological age, weight and anthropometric measures, that weight and age gave the highest multiple correlation with strength as measured by the Roger's Strength Test.

The relation of chronological or skeletal age to performance depends to a great extent upon the range of age included, the sex, and general maturity level of the subjects. Correlation coefficients ranging from .42 to .56 were obtained between seven performance measures and skeletal age of primary school children (Seils, 1951). However, Rarick and Oyster (1964), studying elementary school children, obtained different results in calculating the relationships between chronological age, height, weight, and skeletal age and performance items including the run, standing broad jump, distance throw, and weight strength measures. By holding the maturity measures constant and computing partial correlations for each of the various measures, it was found that neither skeletal age nor any of the other three maturity measures accounted for a major part of the variance in any of the strength or physical performance measures. After further partialling, it was found that chronological age, which gave the highest third order correlation values, accounted for, at most, 15 percent of the variance in strength measures. Rarick and Oyster concluded that skeletal maturity was a factor of little consequence in accounting for individual differences in strength and motor performance, while chronological age was the most important maturity indicator in explaining the variance in strength.

Skeletal maturity is, however, an important factor in superior athletic performance of boys in later childhood. Krogman (1959) reports that of the 55 boys who participated in the 1957 Little League World Series 29 percent had a skeletal age less than their chronological age while 71 percent of the boys had an advanced, or higher skeletal age, in comparison with their chronological age. Similarly, outstanding school athletes, at both the elementary and the junior high school level, were found to have significantly higher skeletal ages than non-athletes (Clarke and Peterson, 1961).

Nonlinearity has been reported in the relationship between age, height, and weight and the athletic events of standing broad jump, softball throw, and six-second run on the basis of tests of 882 boys and 900 girls ranging in age from 9 to 17 years (Cearley, 1957). Actual correlations are very high, however, as would be expected for such a wide age range. When age is held constant, the relationships of a number of physical performance measures to height and to weight are generally low at all ages 10 to 17 for both boys and girls. The relationships of height and weight with various performance items do vary markedly however (Espenschade, 1963).

No significant relationship has been found between performance and body build (Breitinger, 1935; Barry and Cureton, 1961) and body size is not as significant in distinguishing athletes from non-athletes at the elementary school level as it is at the junior high school level (Clarke and Peterson, 1961).

DEVELOPMENT OF STRENGTH

The contraction of the muscles of the body is basic to movement, so that the force with which muscles can contract is of vital interest in a study of motor behavior. If the force of contraction of the muscles is not sufficient to cause movement, the muscle action is isometric and the force so exerted is referred to as static strength while contractions resulting in movement (isotonic muscle action) are referred to as dynamic strength, strength-in-action, or power. Static strength is measured by means of instruments such as the dynamometer and tensiometer which allow no or only extremely limited amounts of movement. Dynamic strength is usually determined by the level of performance in events which measure the ability of the body to develop momentum in propelling external objects or the individual's own body.

Studies of the development of static strength in preschool and elementary school children have usually employed grip strength, as recorded by a hand dynamometer, because of its ease of administration. It is then inferred that such a measure is indicative of general body strength because grip strength has been found to be highly correlated with other static strength measures at older ages (Jones, 1949). Such an assumption may be open to question among younger children.

Metheny (1941a) found there was a rapid gain in grip strength of approximately 65 percent for both boys and girls between the ages of 3 and 6 years. Meredith (1935) noted that boys tend to double their grip strength between the ages of 6 and 11 while an increase of 359 percent is shown between 6 and 18 years of age. A similar study of the grip strength of girls revealed an increase of only 260 percent during the years of 6 to 18 with the discrepancy being largely attributed to their lessened increase in strength during the adolescent years (Metheny, 1941a).

The correlations between grip strength and measures of physical growth such as weight, height, lung capacity, chest girth, and physical vigor for a group of primary and of fourth grade school children led Gates (1924) to conclude that increases in strength are a function of many aspects of growth. Baldwin (1926) and Johnson (1925) have also noted that changes in strength are associated with general growth. Baldwin reports a correlation of .76 between grip strength and chronological age for boys between 7 and 15 years, while Johnson obtained a similar correlation between these same measures from 3 to 13 years. The parallel increases in grip strength and body size were found by Metheny (1941b) to be so close she concluded that the evaluation of grip strength in children should always be considered in the light of the child's body size. A study of the relationship between ankle extensor strength and roentenographic measures of the leg muscles in 51 seven-year-old children produced correlations between these two measures ranging from .58 to .63 for the boys and from .22 to .52 for the girls (Rarick and Thompson, 1956).

Gains in body size reflect the gains made by the various body tissues during growth. Figure 24 indicates that the gains made in bone, muscle, skin, and subcutaneous tissue as recorded by roentenographic measures at the maximum diameter of the calf are fairly consistent during the early part of later childhood. Both sexes show a peak in preadolescent fat increase followed by a negative velocity with the onset of a rapid increase in the development of bone and muscle tissue. In girls this increase and decrease is not as marked as it is in boys, however, and girls tend to maintain a higher level of subcutaneous fat and skin increases. Girls begin to make marked gains in bone and muscle between 9 and 10 years of age while the boys begin their increased gains between 11 and 12 years of age.

When the mean gains in the various body tissues are compared with the isometric strength means of various muscle groups from ages 7 to 12 years (Table 10) similarities in gains may be observed.

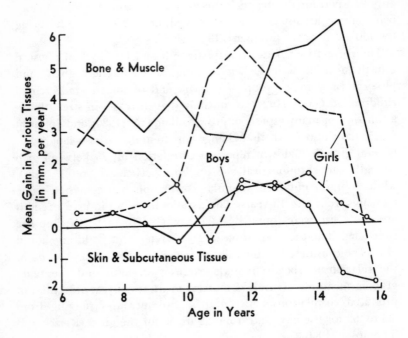

Figure 24.   Gains in breadth of bone, muscle, skin and subcutaneous tissue. (Adapted from data by O. M. Lombard, "Breadth of Bone and Muscle by Age and Sex in Childhood." **Child Develpm.**, 21:229-239, 1950.)

The mean strength scores in Table 10 are based upon the data of 115 boys and 101 girls who were tested in the Elementary School Growth Study conducted in Madison, Wisconsin, under the direction of members of the Department of Physical Education of the University of Wisconsin. It is interesting to note that the greatest

Table 10

Isometric Strength Means for Various Muscle Groups†
(in pounds)

Age (years)	7	8	9	10	11	12
Ankle Extensor						
Boys	60	67.5	83.5	89.5	96 *	123.5
Girls	56.5	66.5	75.5*	96.5	101.5	102
Knee Extensor						
Boys	63.5	75	96.5	107.5	110.5*	151.5
Girls	64.5	76.5	83.5*	116.5	127.5	139.5
Hip Extensors						
Boys	40.5	46.5	58	59.5	65.5*	87.5
Girls	34.5	44.5	47	57.5	63.5	73
Elbow Flexors						
Boys	31.5	41.5	45	50.5	56.5*	67.5
Girls	31	35.5	41 *	50.5	50.5	56.5
Shoulder Adductors						
Boys	37	49	53	53.5	64 *	81
Girls	33.5	43.5	43.5*	55.5	56	59
Shoulder Medial Rotators						
Boys	20	25.5	27.5	28	31.5*	37.5
Girls	16.5	21	22.5	25.5	28.5	29
Wrist flexors						
Boys	23	25.5	29.5	32.5	33 *	42
Girls	20.5	22	25	28.5	29.5*	39

* Start of period of greatest gain

† The authors are indebted to Professor G. L. Rarick, University of Wisconsin, for permission to use these data.

gains in the strength made by the girls in four of the strength measures occur between 9 and 10 years while the boys make their greatest gains in strength in seven of the strength measures between 11 and 12 years of age.

It is possible that variations occur with respect to the onset of the greatest amount of gain in the various muscle groupings. Table 10 indicates both girls and boys make the greatest gain in wrist flexors between 11 and 12 years, whereas there is a difference of 2 years in the onset of gains in other muscle groupings for the sexes. In close association with wrist flexors, right grip strength shows its most marked gain for a group of California girls between the ages of 10 and 11 years to bring the mean right grip strength of the girls to the same value as that of the boys (Keogh, 1965).

Although the girls equal, or even surpass, the boys in strength at the peak of girls' strength gains, there is a definite sex difference in the strength of elementary school children (Metheny, 1941b; Rarick and Thompson, 1956; Keogh, 1965). Boys are found to be substantially stronger and, on the average, possess the greater muscle size. The degree of sex difference in strength attributable to androgen production in the male during preadolescence would appear to be negligible, since equating boys and girls on the basis of muscle size reveals a superiority in strength for the boys which is significant only at the 30 percent level of confidence (Rarick and Thompson, 1956).

Even though increases in strength accompany increases in body size, Meredith (1935) noted that the coefficient of variation in strength was, with the exception of weight, two to five times as great as any of the 18 anthropometric measures used in the University of Iowa Studies in Child Welfare. The greatest variabilities in strength were found to occur during periods of rapid developmental change, and growth in strength was noted to be less variable in childhood than during pubescence and post-pubescence. Similarly, the coefficient of variation for measurements of the breadth of bone and muscle tissue is around the level of 8 percent until 10 years of age, when the variation increases markedly for the girls in conjunction with the prepubertal growth spurt noted in Figure 24. An increase in variation also occurs for the boys in association with the marked increases in bone and muscle tissue at 12 years (Lombard, 1950).

The tendency for girls to be more variable in measurements of breadth of bone and muscle tissue even during the relatively stable period of childhood, may, in part, account for the lower correlation coefficients obtained by Rarick and Thompson (1956) of the relationship between ankle extensor strength and muscle breadth in girls.

The development of muscular strength is symmetrical on both sides of the body with strength being slightly greater on the dominant side of the body. Similarly, the percentage contributed to total strength by the arms and the legs tends to remain consistent between the ages of 5 to 18 years, with the legs contributing approximately 60 percent to total strength (Martin, 1918). Such findings are in keeping with a relatively symmetrical body structure and the greater muscle mass in the leg area in comparison with the musculature of the arms.

The relationship between static and dynamic strength has challenged a large number of investigators but, in general, little relationship has been obtained between static strength and motor performance in specific activities. Where relatively high relationships have been found these have usually involved multiple correlations of a number of events. Carpenter's study (1942b) of the relationship between static dynamometric strength of the shoulder girdle muscles and certain motor performance events is typical of this type of approach. Using as subjects 217 primary grade boys and girls, this investigator obtained a multiple correlation of .50 for girls and .63 for boys when correlating "total shoulder girdle strength," (the sum of right grip, left grip, pull, and push), with weight and performance in the broad jump and shot-put. On the basis of her results, she calculated the following regression equations as predictive of total strength for primary school children:

Boys' Strength = .1 broad jump + 2.3 shot-put + weight
Girls' Strength = .5 broad jump + 3.0 shot-put + weight.

As a confirmation of her results, Carpenter (1942a) correlated the two dynamic strength measures in her regression equation with a composite score of the motor performance of primary school children in eight track and field events. The correlations between the motor performance total points score and the two dynamic strength measures were .70 for both the broad jump and the shot-put for boys, and .74 for the broad jump and .61 for the shot-put for the girls. Although these correlation coefficients indicate a substantial relationship between the dynamic strength measures as defined by Carpenter and a total points score of performance in events commonly engaged in by children of this age, it by no means indicates any relationship between static and dynamic strength. However, the shot-put may be considered a good predictor of dynamic strength in the arms and the broad jump a good predictor of dynamic strength in the legs. Moreover, as the relative distribution of strength appears to have a consistent development (Martin, 1918), either one could be expected to be a reasonably good predictor of general dynamic strength.

Some significant correlations have been obtained between static strength and performance in specific activities, however. In relating the static strength of leg extensor muscle groups in 100 elementary school girls to the distance covered in the standing broad jump, Barsanti (1954) obtained significant correlations of .35 between the knee extensors and the standing broad jump and of .24 between the hip extensors and performance in the same activity. An exploration of the relationship between propulsive force and various leg extensor strengths in 10 boys at ages 8, 10, and 12 years resulted in correlation coefficients approaching the significance level at 10 and 12 years with only one value, of .64 for the hip strength at 10 years, actually being significant at the 5 percent level (Eckert, 1964).

Acceleration is a component of propulsive force so it is not surprising that correlations ranging from .52 to .73 were found for the relationship between static hip extensor strength and speed of angular movement in the hip joint (Eckert, 1964). Subsequently, higher values ranging from .74 to .79 have been found between static strength and speed of arm movement (Nelson & Fahrney, 1965). It is possible that when activities are analyzed in terms of the amount of force or energy required for their execution that a substantial relationship will be found to exist between static and dynamic strength (Eckert, 1965). An unpublished study on college women (Eckert and Day) in which a correlation coefficient of .76 was obtained for the relationship between pushing arm strength and total work load in doing push-ups indicates a further possibility of a substantial relationship between static strength and motor performance in events of short duration.

CHANGES IN MOTOR PERFORMANCE

With the steady increments that have been noted in body size and in strength, it is to be expected that there are also consistent increments in the basic skills of running, jumping, and throwing during later childhood. Similarly, the slight differences that have been noted favoring boys in these areas are duplicated in slightly better performances in running and jumping for boys. Distance throwing, however, shows an increasingly marked sex difference after the age of 5 years. Figures 25 through 28, based upon averages compiled from the data of a number of investigators, illustrate the changes with age in these activities for boys and girls from 5 to 17 years.

a. Running. The speed with which an individual can run depends upon the length of the stride as well as its tempo. Figure 25 shows that there is a steady increase in running speed during the period of early childhood which can easily be explained in terms of the steady increase in body size with its concomitant increases in lever length and strength providing increased length and tempo to the running stride. It is also, in part, a reflection of an increase in ability to run greater distances with increasing age. It is quite obvious that the start in the run has less effect on the total time of the dash in longer runs than in shorter runs. Therefore, in calculations based upon yards per second, the older age groupings, which tend to be based upon 50 and 60 yard dashes, have a lesser starting time influence in their yards-per-second averages than do the younger age groupings where the runs are usually 30 to 35 yards in length.

b. Jumping. The increases with age in both a vertical jump and a jump for distance are shown in Figures 26 and 27 respectively. Increases in body size with age have both advantageous and detrimental effects upon performance in jumping. The increased body weight that occurs with increases in lever length and muscle mass must be overcome by proportionately greater gains accruing from these increments. Improvements in the mechanics involved in jump-

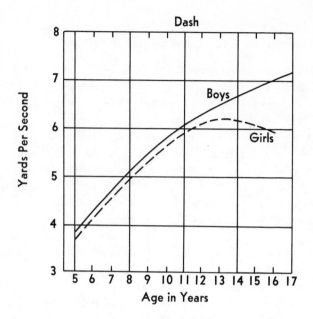

Figure 25.   Running. (From **Science and Medicine of Exercise and Sports,** edited by Warren R. Johnson: Copyright © 1960 by Warren R. Johnson: "Motor Development" by Anna Espenschade. Reprinted by permission of Harper & Row, Publishers.)

ing would also appear to be a contributing factor to increases in performance.

An extensive investigation of the cinematographic records of six poor, average, and good jumpers of both sexes at each level from 6 to 12 years revealed that earlier thigh flexion appears as a sex difference after the age of 9 when the boys exhibit this characteristic sooner than the girls at all levels of performance (Clayton, 1936). A similar sex difference appears with respect to earlier trunk flexion for the boys at all performance levels from 9 through 12 years. Clayton concludes that there is some evidence of sequential

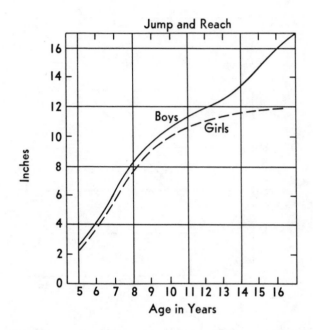

Figure 26.   Jump and reach. (From **Science and Medicine of Exercise and Sports,** edited by Warren R. Johnson: Copyright © 1960 by Warren R. Johnson: "Motor Development" by Anna Espenschade. Reprinted by permission of Harper & Row, Publishers.)

development in the mechanics of the standing broad jump in children from 9 to 12 years of age, with boys in particular progressing toward a more mature and efficient manner of jumping.

It is not surprising, therefore, that jumping has been considered a predictor of body strength (Carpenter, 1942b) and also a diagnostic test of motor coordination. Cowan and Pratt (1934) tested 540 children ranging in age from 3 to 12 years in their ability to hurdle jump and then plotted curves of growth in skill at successively higher age levels using median and Gesell "C" scores. Both these methods showed a continuous and relatively gradual improvement

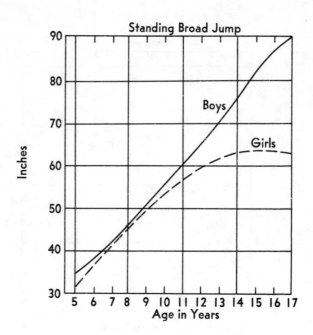

Figure 27.   Standing broad jump. (From **Science and Medicine of Exercise and Sports,** edited by Warren R. Johnson: Copyright © 1960 by Warren R. Johnson: "Motor Development" by Anna Espenschade. Reprinted by permission of Harper & Row, Publishers.)

in hurdle jumping over the entire age range, with there being a slight indication of a sex difference in favor of girls below 7 years and of boys above this age level. Cowan and Pratt obtained no relationship between performance level at any age period and height or weight. They did, however, obtain a raw correlation of .77 between jumping performance and chronological age. As the correlation between age and the jump was .57 with height and weight partialled out, these investigators concluded that maturation was the determining factor influencing the height of the hurdle jump and, as such, the hurdle jump is a true developmental test of motor coordination. However, another study of the relationship between the hurdle jump and performance in the standing broad jump, the jump and reach, the distance throw, and the 35 yard dash resulted in correlation coefficients ranging from .44 to .53 (Hartman, 1943). Since similar intercorrelations of the order of .50 among the comparative events were also obtained, it was concluded that the hurdle jump could be considered no better measure of general motor proficiency than any of the other measures.

In general, performance in jumping has been found to improve with advancing age, with the degree of improvement being greater for boys than for girls. However, there is a large variability in performance which results in considerable overlapping of performance scores between age groups and sexes. Kane and Meredith (1952) noted that the average jumpers at 7 years jumped approximately as far as the poorer ten percent of 11 year olds. Furthermore, the performances of the upper ten percent of the 9 year olds were equal or superior to the performance level of the middle 40 percent of the 11 year olds. Since these findings are based upon cross-sectional data, one may speculate as to whether some of this variability may be caused by differential growth rates. However, Glassow and Kruse (1960), reporting on the motor performance of 123 girls, aged 6 through 14 years, for whom data were available for at least three consecutive years, noted that individuals tended to remain in the same relative position within the group during the elementary school years; this being especially so in the run and the standing broad jump.

The maintenance of an individual's position in a group with respect to performance level in jumping may be as much a factor of mechanical execution as it would appear to be of body size. Cinematographical analyses of ten skilled and ten non-skilled performances in the standing broad jump indicate that there are characteristic differences in the angles of take-off and of landing and in the extent and duration of specific joint actions (Zimmerman, 1956). Skilled performers employ a greater range of movement in their performances with a greater amount of hip and knee flexion as the legs are drawn up under the body. There are also greater amounts of hip, knee, and ankle extension during the propulsive phase of the jump.

c. **Throwing.** The development of throwing ability is usually measured by the distance variously sized balls can be thrown and the increasing ability with chronological age in this type of throw is illustrated in Figure 28. It is quite obvious that boys tend to be greatly superior to girls in the distance throw at all age levels and that this difference becomes increasingly great with increases in age. Wild's previously reported observations (1938) of the development of the overhand throwing pattern would indicate that some of this difference is caused by less mature throwing patterns on the part of girls. The larger forearm length and girth noted in boys also gives them a mechanical and strength advantage in the propulsion of an object for distance. Throws for accuracy, where production of force is not so demanding, since distance is confined along with the target area, do not produce such marked sex differences. However, such a difference does exist favoring the boys and here also there is improvement in performance with increasing age (Keogh, 1965).

d. **Flexibility.** Studies of flexibility have usually been conducted in conjunction with other aspects of motor performance and few have been concerned with age differences during the school years. However, one such study was undertaken by Hupprich and Sigerseth (1950) where twelve measures of flexibility were taken on 300 girls ranging in age from 6 to 18 years. There was a general increase in flexibility until the girls approached the age of 12 years, with a general decline thereafter. Exceptions to this trend were found in the shoulder, knee, and thigh where the girls showed a consistent decline in flexibility from 6 to 18 years. Eighteen-year-old girls were more flexible in certain aspects of five measurements than were girls 6 years of age. Of all the measures, ankle flexibility appeared to be the most constant throughout all the age groups and varied no more than 2.94 degrees at any age. Analysis of the results revealed low intercorrelations between the twelve measures of flexibility, which strongly suggests that a general flexibility factor does not exist and that each major joint appears to have its own specific flexibility. In this latter regard, it was noted that not a single girl was significantly above the average nor significantly below the average in all twelve measurements while only six of the 300 girls reached their respective age-group averages in all twelve measurements.

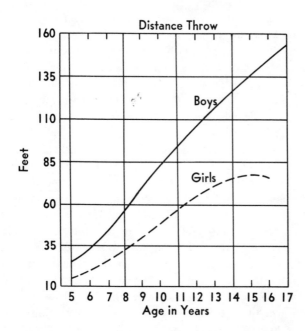

Figure 28.   Distance throw. (From **Science and Medicine of Exercise and Sports,** edited by Warren R. Johnson: Copyright © 1960 by Warren R. Johnson: "Motor Development" by Anna Espenschade. Reprinted by permission of Harper & Row, Publishers.)

   e. **Balance.** From the previous discussions of the various large muscle activities, it is obvious that varying degrees of balance are required for successful performance. Two distinct types of balance have been identified as operating in most of our daily activities; namely, dynamic and static balance (Seashore, 1947; McCloy, 1945). The maintenance of a particular body position with a minimum of sway is referred to as static balance while dynamic balance is considered to be the maintenance of posture during the performance of a motor skill which tends to disturb the body's orientation. The distinct nature of these two types of balance is revealed by the low correlation of .34 obtained by Bass (1939) between measures of static and dynamic balance.

Walking board tests to measure dynamic balance were first standardized by Seashore (1947) and he reported steady improvements in boys from 5 to 11 years with a subsequent leveling off until 18 years. Similarly, steady improvement in both sexes of ages 5 through 11 is reported by Wallon et al. (1958) on the basis of different walking board tests. On the basis of railwalking tests given to over 700 Philadelphia children ranging in age from 6 to 14, continuing improvement for both sexes is reported over the entire age range studied although there is some suggestion of a slackening in rate of gain from 12 to 14, especially for females (Heath, 1949). A repeat of this study over the age range of 8 to 16 years reports essentially the same results, including showing a slackening in rate of growth in females from 12 to 14 years (Goetzinger, 1961).

However, Keogh (1965) claims there is rather clear indication that performance in beam walking does not increase steadily with age during childhood. He finds a consistent age change in boys except for a leveling off from 7 to 9 whereas girls have a marked increase from 7 to 8 followed by a leveling off from 8 to 10. An examination of the results of Seashore, Heath, Goetzinger, and his own lead Keogh to the conclusion that mean age performance in beam walking remains stable for several years followed by a marked increase. Exact identification of the ages where the increases occur is not attempted but it is suggested that they seem to be somewhere between 6 and 8 and between 9 and 11 with a plateau in performance between these increases. A comparison of these results with previously noted periods of rapid increments and plateaus in the development of bone and muscle tissue and of strength does not reveal a consistent patterning but there is some suggestion that the plateaus in balance may coincide with the increments in bone and muscle tissue and in strength, with the reverse situation occurring with increments in balance. Certainly, a longitudinal study of all these factors would shed much more light on their interrelationships than the cross-sectional data that are currently available.

Sex differences in dynamic balance are reported by both Heath (1949) and Goetzinger (1961) favoring greater improvement in boys whereas Keogh (1965) obtained sex differences during the periods of increase but none during the plateaus. Great variability has been found to exist among the levels of performance within a particular age group; for example, Seashore (1947) noted that some 7-year-olds were equal in performance to the average 15-year-olds while the poorest 14-year-olds were at the level of the lowest quarter of 7-year-olds.

A static balance test in which the subjects were timed as to their ability to remain on a balance stick, 1″ x 1″ x 12″, when the foot was placed lengthwise on the long axis of the stick was used by Seils (1951) to determine level of performance in children of the first three grades. Analysis of the data indicated a rather constant increase between 6 and 8 years. Static balance on a beam reveals age spurts for girls over the period 5 to 11 years whereas boys show a more consistent increase over the same age span (Keogh, 1965). Starting at the age of 6, steady increases are reported in the pre-pubescent years for both boys and girls in performance on the stabilometer (Bachman, 1961).

No sex differences are reported in studies of static balance. However, variability is again reported to be great within any one age level (Seils, 1951). Some of the investigators suggest that the similarity in results between dynamic and static balance indicate a probability that growth in both may follow a similar course (Seils, 1951; Keogh, 1965). Furthermore, the wide range of proficiency in balancing activities at each age level seems to suggest that selective factors may be operating with respect to such proficiency and the choice of general motor activities made by children.

f. Coordination. An individual is said to show good coordination when he moves easily and the sequence and timing of his acts are well controlled. This essential element of motor performance is not readily measured objectively although high achievement in any event implies good coordination. Good general coordination should then be reflected in high achievement in a number of activities. A glance at the intercorrelations reported by various investigators of the relationships among the basic skills of running, jumping, and throwing indicates little communality (Table 11). No consistent trends are evidenced although there does seem to be a tendency for relationships between the dash and broad jump and between the broad jump and distance throw for boys to be slightly higher at

Table 11

Intercorrelations Reported by Various Investigators*

Age	Dash with Broad Jump		Dash with Distance Throw	
	Boys	Girls	Boys	Girls
49-78 mo.		.53		.36
1st 3 grades	.475	.576	.244	.442
10-14 yr.		.61		.43
10-13 yr.	.665		.502	
Jr. H.S.	.642		.545	
	.787			
	.64	.61	.38	.51
	.67	.64	.48	.44
Sr. H.S.	.44			
	.76			
	.58	.60		
	.48	.45	.38	.41
	.49		.24	.23
		.57		

Age	Broad Jump and Distance Throw		Broad Jump with Jump and Reach	
	Boys	Girls	Boys	Girls
49-78 mo.		.41		.53
1st 3 grades	.311	.441	.401	.547
8 year	.58	.35	.63	.62
10-13 yr.	.53			
10-14 yr.				.49
Jr. H.S.	.721			
	.39	.45	.42	.30
	.60	.51	.45	.37
Sr. H.S.	.46	.48	.65	.56
	.47	.42	.51	.64
			.604	

* From *Science and Medicine of Exercise and Sports*, edited by Warren R. Johnson: Copyright © 1960 by Warren R. Johnson: "Motor Development" by Anna Espenschade. Reprinted by permission of Harper & Row, Publishers.

the junior high school level than either before or after this time. In the case of girls, however, correlations are of approximately the same order at all age levels.

With such low intercorrelations being found between the basic motor activities, it is not surprising that attempts have been made to measure coordination with special coordination tests. The most commonly used test of coordination is the Brace test with its graded series of 20 stunts. Although an attempt was made to select events which measure control, balance, agility, and flexibility, and to provide for even steps in difficulty, these aims have been imperfectly met. One of its drawbacks is the scoring of all items on a pass or fail basis. As some individuals can pass all tests in the battery, the range is also inadequate for all abilities. However, the test is fairly objective and reliable and has been shown to measure abilities which are only slightly, if at all, related to strength and height or weight.

Both sexes perform equally well and consistently improve in total performance in the Brace test until the age of 11 years, after which there is an increasingly greater sex difference, with girls leveling off while boys continue to improve at a relatively consistent rate (Figure 29). The percentage of both sexes passing the items designated as measuring "control" and "agility" is approximately equal between 10.5 and 13 years (Espenschade, 1947). The most striking sex difference at all ages is item five of the Brace test consisting of 3 push-ups, while the greatest similarity is in item 7 where the individual sits down and then stands again with the arms folded and the feet crossed.

When various test items of motor coordination are subjected to factor analysis, there would seem to be a considerable amount of interrelationship between balance, speed, agility, and control which tends to be task-specific. For example, administration of 23 items that had been used to measure some phase of motor coordination to 92 third and fourth grade girls produced, when the data were subjected to the multiple-group method of factoring, nine factors (Cumbee et al., 1957). Five of the nine factors extracted were identified as: balancing objects; total body quick change of direction; speed of change of direction of arms and hands; body balance; and vertical total body quick change of direction. The results obtained

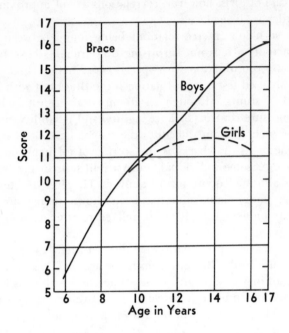

Figure 29.   Brace test. (From **Science and Medicine of Exercise and Sports,** edited by Warren R. Johnson: Copyright © 1960 by Warren R. Johnson: "Motor Development" by Anna Espenschade. Reprinted by permission of Harper & Row, Publishers.)

in this study were compared with a similar factor analysis of motor coordinations of women at the college level (Cumbee, 1954) with the variable findings suggesting that consideration should be given to a different definition of motor coordination for different age levels.

g. **General.** Innumerable studies have been undertaken of various specific motor performances, while others have attempted to develop some index based upon performance in specific activities which would give an over-all rating or predict general motor ability, educability, agility, or coordination. In addition to the motor activities already mentioned, these have included such things as grasping, striking, relaying objects, catching, kicking, hopping, and various quick changes in body position. These activities have all been found to show increased performance with age in varying degrees of increment for boys and girls.

In general, boys have been found to excel in those activities requiring strength and in grosser movements, whereas girls tend to excel in the finer coordination activities such as exactness in walking, speed in grasping, exactness of grasping, and lying down (Yarmolenko, 1933). Girls have been found to be superior to boys in performance in the 50 foot hop in one instance (Jenkins, 1930) whereas in other instances mean performance in the same test has been found to be almost identical for both sexes during childhood (Meyer, 1951; Keogh, 1965). In all of the studies, however, a greater percentage of boys failed to complete the entire fifty foot distance of the test and, in controlled hopping, girls were found to be superior to boys at ages from 6 through 9 (Keogh, 1965). In the latter instance, girls were more graceful and hopped on the balls of their feet whereas boys hopped in a very flat-footed manner. Differences were also noted in the technique of good and poor performers. The less able children held their non-hopping foot in a high position with the knee and foot in front of the body rather than down and behind the body in a lower position as is done by more able performers (Keogh, 1965).

Boys have been found to be superior to girls in kicking a ball for distance with the superiority of the boys increasing with advancing age as it does in the distance throw (Jenkins, 1930; Yarmolenko, 1933).

In the majority of activities at all age levels, however, there is a great deal of variability in performance, so that there is a considerable overlapping of the sexes in performance within a given age level (Jenkins, 1930). Children are still perfecting their skills and some of the variability is undoubtedly due to the propensity to avoid repetition of combinations of movements that have produced unsuccessful results (Victors, 1961).

INTEREST AND MOTOR ACTIVITY

It is to be expected that there will be varying degrees of interest in motor activity among children as there is among adults. To a large extent such interest will depend upon the opportunities for motor activity and the interest that is expressed in such activity by the persons with whom the child identifies during the growing years. Interest has been found to increase in motor activities through childhood to adolescence, with a marked increase during the latter part of childhood and early adolescence for both boys and girls (Figures 30 and 31). This is, of course, the period in which the child wants to be a member of the "gang" and motor activities offer an excellent opportunity for such association.

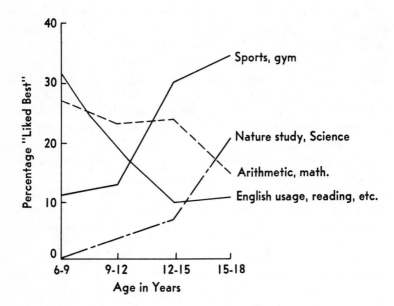

Figure 30.   Expressed interests of boys. (From data by A. T. Jersild and R. Tasch, **Children's Interests and What They Suggest for Education.** New York: Bureau of Publications, Teachers College, Columbia University, 1949. By permission of the publisher.)

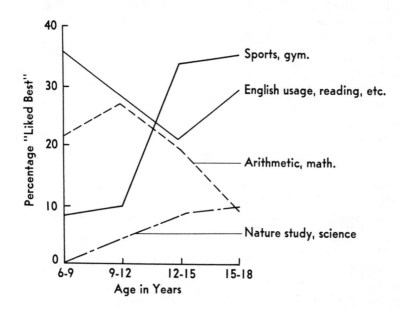

Figure 31.   Expressed interests of girls. (From data by
               A. T. Jersild and R. Tasch, **Children's Inter-
               ests and What They Suggest for Education.**
               New York: Bureau of Publications, Teachers
               College, Columbia University, 1949. By per-
               mission of the publisher.)

After 9 years of age the child begins to perfect an increasing
number of activities which will enable him to take part in adult
sports and games with only body size limiting the level of performance. Such emulation of adult activities undoubtedly is a factor
in increasing interest. Conversely, however, lack of ability will also
be a deterrent at this peer-conscious age and will result in withdrawal from unproficient areas and an expressed decline in interest.

More proficient children have been found to come from homes
where the parents have been highly active in sports and have pro-

vided the children with greater opportunity and provision for play. These included a wider variety of play materials at an earlier age which allowed for the use of large muscle activity and more frequent visitations to playgrounds so that the child acquired a wider range of interests and activity in play (Rarick and McKee, 1949). Opportunities for participation in good physical education programs in school also contribute to proficiency. A comparison of 81 twelve-year-old boys who had participated in a good physical education program for at least three years was made with 81 boys of the same age who had had little or no physical education in the elementary school. Although the two groups were similar with respect to chronological age, weight, height, skeletal age, and Wetzel grid developmental level, the boys in the good program surpassed the boys in the poor program in the Rogers Physical Fitness Index, the Metheny-Johnson Test of Motor Educability, the Indiana Fitness Test, the vertical jump, and back, leg, and arm strength (Whittle, 1961).

Opportunities for the perfecting of the skills that have been developed during infancy and early childhood remain of considerable importance in later childhood if the child is to maintain a level of performance similar to his age-mates.

CHAPTER IX

ADOLESCENT DEVELOPMENT

Adolescence is usually said to begin with the physical changes relating to puberty and to continue until growth is complete and the individual thus is mature, in a physical sense. The biologically most important of these is the development of the reproductive system into its mature state in both sexes. Figure 32, illustrating the growth in weight of the testes, prostate, ovaries, and uterus, shows that the development of the reproductive organs begins earlier in females than in males. The onset of puberty is difficult to assess in males and is usually based upon the development of the secondary sex characteristics and the growth of the genitalia. In females, the menarche, or first menstrual period, is usually taken as the onset of puberty although Ashley Montagu (1946) has pointed out that the adolescent girl may be sterile for some months after the onset of menstruation.

In boys, the first sign of impending puberty is usually an acceleration in the growth of the testes and scrotum with, perhaps, slight growth in pubic hair beginning at same time. Pubic hair

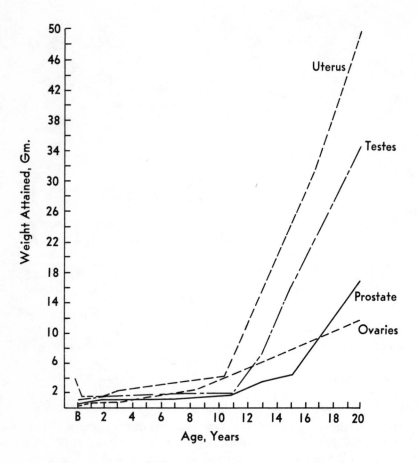

Figure 32.   Growth in weight of the reproductive organs.
(From J. M. Tanner, **Growth at Adolescence.**
Oxford, Eng.: Blackwell Scientific Publica-
tions, 1955. By permission of the publisher.)

growth tends to proceed slowly until the beginning of the general
growth spurt, after which it increases rapidly to its mature distribution. In general, the spurts in height and penis growth begin
about a year after the onset of testicular acceleration. Although

this sequence of events tends to be relatively consistent in the development of boys, the times at which they occur is extremely variable so that it is possible to have boys at the ages of 13 and 14 years who may vary in development from childhood through all stages to almost complete maturity. Figure 33, developed by Tanner (1955) from the data presented in numerous studies of adolescent males, indicates the timing of these developmental events for an average boy and also the range of ages at which each event may begin and reach its termination.

For girls, the first sign of approaching puberty is usually the appearance of the breast bud, although the appearance of pubic hair may sometimes precede it. Figure 34, also developed by Tanner (1955) from the data presented in a number of studies of adolescent girls, shows the sequence of events for the average girl with the range in times for the appearance of breast bud, beginning of pubic hair growth, menarche, and peak velocity in height being indicated directly under each event. It may be noted that the range and duration of the events associated with adolescence in females appears to be less than those characteristic of males during adolescence.

A number of scales are available for rating genital developmental stages, breast development stages, and pubic hair stages. Typical of the first is the following five stage rating of genitalia maturation in males:

(1) Infantile; (2) enlargement of scrotum, first reddening and texture change; (3) first "sculpturing" and enlargement of penis; (4) pronounced sculpturing and darkening; (5) essentially adult; reddish brown color, loose penile skin, loss of sharp sculpturing.*

A five stage rating scale for female breast development is as follows:

(1) The infantile form: elevation of papilla only; (2) the bud stage: elevation of the breast and papilla as a small mound; (3) inter-

* From E. L. Reynolds & J. V. Wines, "Physical changes associated with adolescence in boys." *Amer. J. Dis. Child.*, 82:529-547, 1951. By permission of the authors and publisher.

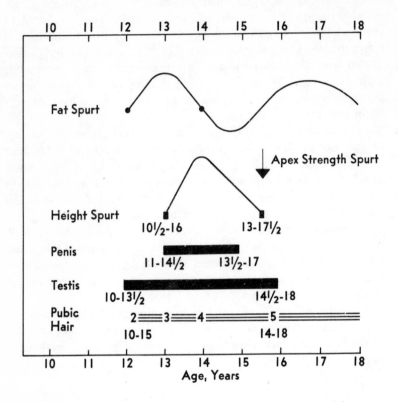

Figure 33.   Diagram of sequence of events at adoles-
                cence in boys. An average boy is repre-
                sented: the range of ages within which each
                event charted may begin and end is given by
                the figures placed directly below its start
                and finish. (From J. M. Tanner, **Growth at
                Adolescence.** Oxford, Eng.: Blackwell Scien-
                tific Publications, 1955. By permission of the
                publisher.)

mediate stage: elevation of breast and areola with no distinct separa-
tion of their contours; (4) primary mamma stage; areola and papilla
form a secondary mound above the level of the breast; (5) mature

stage; the papilla only projects, owing to the recession of the areola to the general contour of the breast.*

The development of pubic hair in boys has also been classified into five stages, namely:

(1) Infantile; (2) first appearance, pigmented, usually straight, sparse; (3) slight curl, slight spread, usually darker; (4) curled, moderate amount and spread, not yet extended to thighs; (5) "adult" in type, profuse, forming an inverse triangle extending to thighs.**

Although pubic hair rating stages differ from those of genitalia and breast development, they are the most frequently used to assess sexual development, since they are most reliably observed. Axillary hair generally appears about two years after the beginning of pubic hair growth which places it at approximately the end of pubic hair stage 3. In boys, facial hair begins to grow at about the time that axillary hair first appears and its development is usually not completed until stage 5 is reached in both pubic hair and genitalia development. The remainder of the body hair in males starts to appear at this time also and continues to do so for a considerable time afterwards, with the hair on the thigh, calf, abdomen, and forearm usually preceding that on the chest and upper arms.

Other secondary sex changes include the enlargement of the larynx in boys, which tends to coincide with the spurt in sitting height, and the deepening of the voice. Both sexes have an increase in axillary sweating, which is believed to be due to an enlargement of the apocrine sweat glands of the axilla that begins at approximately the time of axillary hair growth (Tanner, 1955). Intercorrelations which have been calculated to determine the relationships between the various criteria of maturity produce corre-

---

* From E. L. Reynolds & J. V. Wines, "Individual differences in physical changes associated with adolescence in girls." *Amer. J. Dis. Child.*, 75:329-350, 1948. By permission of the authors and publisher.
** From E. L. Reynolds & J. V. Wines, "Physical changes associated with adolescence in boys." *Amer. J. Dis. Child.*, 82:529-547, 1951. By permission of the authors and publisher.

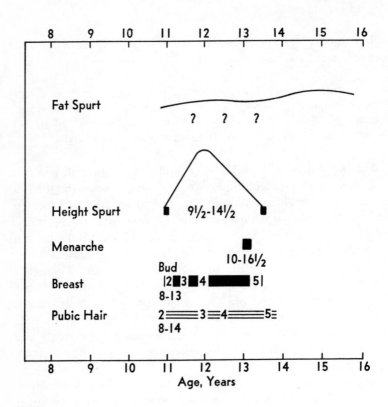

Figure 34.   Diagram of sequence of events at adolescence in girls. An average girl is represented: the range of ages within which some of the events may occur is given by the figures placed directly below them. (From J. M. Tanner, **Growth at Adolescence.** Oxford, Eng.: Blackwell Scientific Publications, 1955. By permission of the publisher.)

lation coefficients ranging from .71 to .95 (Nicolson and Hanley, 1953) indicating there is a unity in the adolescent spurt with respect to bodily growth, physiological changes, and growth of the reproductive organs.

FACTORS AFFECTING THE ONSET OF PUBERTY

Since the menarche in girls is an easily ascertained event, its occurrence is usually used to study trends in the onset of puberty. A marked secular trend of lowering in the age of menarche has been noted (Mills, 1950). Figure 35 indicates the average ages at menarche from 1850 to 1950 in Norway and over segments of this period for girls in Sweden, Finland, and at a women's college in the United States. It is interesting to note that the trend is very similar in all these areas with the menarche occurring $\frac{1}{3}$ to $\frac{1}{2}$ year earlier per decade between the period of 1850 to 1950.

Figure 35 also indicates that there are age differences in the onset of menarche in the various countries. On the basis of a number of studies, it would appear that these regional variations in the menarche tend to be caused by climatic, nutritional, and racial differences. A survey of the average age at first menstruation for girls in the Americas, Europe, and Asia indicates that the menarche occurs consistently earlier in the central temperate areas and tends to be delayed in the colder northern and southern regions. The menarche also appears earlier in girls in the United States than in any other country (Shuttleworth, 1949). Mills (1950) found that prolonged heat tended to retard growth in girls and delay the onset of menarche whereas boys did not show as great a susceptibility to heat. Similar results were obtained by Ellis (1950) in comparing a group of Nigerian school children with a control group of school children in Great Britain.

Little or no difference between the average ages of sexual maturity in Negro and white boys is reported (Ramsey, 1950). Ito (1942), however, reports varying ages of menarche for girls of different racial origin who were attending Los Angeles City College. Those girls of Mexican origin had an average menarcheal age of 12.5, for Europeans it was 12.9, while for Japanese and Negroes it was 13.1 and for Chinese 13.9 years. Conversely, no difference is reported in the age of menarche between whites and Negroes of similar economic circumstances in New York (Michelson, 1944). Certainly racial differences do exist, since there is a marked similarity in the age of menarche among members of a family (Krogman, 1948).

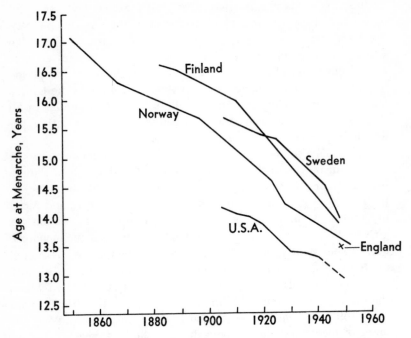

Figure 35.   Secular trend in age at menarche, 1850 to 1950. (From J. M. Tanner, **Growth at Adolescence.** Oxford, Eng.: Blackwell Scientific Publications. By permission of the publisher.)

Differences within racial groupings also exist either as natural variation or on a nutritional basis. Bolk (1926) and Ley (1938) noted that in both Amsterdam and Mainz darker-haired children tended to have a later menarche whereas the reverse situation might be expected on the grounds that the hair tends to darken somewhat with age. The menarche was found to occur 1.6 years sooner in school girls in Columbo, Ceylon, than in girls of rural areas of the same country (Wilson and Sutherland, 1953). The influence of nutrition is pointed up by Ito's data (1942) which shows that Japanese girls born and reared in California mature 1½ years earlier than those born in California but reared in Japan.

FACTORS AFFECTING PUBERAL GROWTH SPURT

A comparison of the appearance of the puberal height spurt in both boys and girls of Sweden as measured in 1883 and in 1938 reveals a trend toward acceleration of the growth spurt in keeping with the previously reported earlier appearance of the menarche (Broman et al., 1942). Figure 36 illustrates this secular trend in the adolescent growth spurt. Boys have a large displacement in the peak of gain, and the amount of growth in height is greater for both sexes during preadolescence in the 1938 children. Other data indicate that the peak height gain occurred as late as age 17 in males in the year 1800 (Kiil, 1939) in comparison with current data which places the peak gain in height between 14 and 15 years in boys.

The marked tendency for puberty to occur earlier as indicated by the foregoing studies of the menarche and of the growth spurt has led to speculation as to causative influences. Mills (1949) has theorized that the acceleration in growth is due to a gradual change in world temperature conditions and cites as evidence work with experimental animals indicating that conditions which create difficulty of heat loss tend to retard growth. Most investigators, however, usually credit better nutrition and generally improved environmental circumstances for the secular trend toward earlier maturation and cite the slowing down of growth and the retardation of puberty during malnutrition. The data of Howe and Schiller (1952) indicate a uniform increase in the heights and weights of school children of all ages in Stuttgart, Germany, for the period from 1920 to 1940, with a reversal during the latter part of the 1939-1945 war period when the food intake of the children was considerably restricted. From additional data collected in France by Douady and Tremolieres (1947) and in Belgium by Ellis (1945) it appears that war-time privation may be more effective in retarding puberty than in slowing down earlier growth.

Numerous studies indicate that during short periods of malnutrition the organism's growth is slowed up as if to wait for better times. When conditions improve, growth takes place unusually rapidly until the animal has returned to its genetically determined growth curve and growth again proceeds at its normal rate (Clarke and Smith, 1938; Barnes et al., 1947). On the basis of data collected

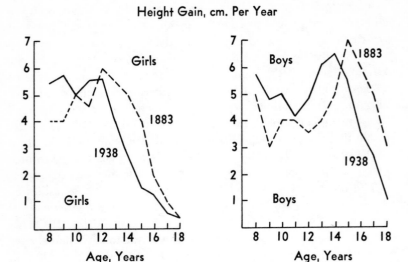

Height Gain, cm. Per Year

Figure 36. Secular trend in time of adolescent spurt. Velocity curves of height for Swedish girls and boys measured in 1883 and 1938/39. (From J. M. Tanner, **Growth at Adolescence.** Oxford, Eng.: Blackwell Scientific Publications, 1955. By permission of the publisher.)

by Engle et al. (1937) on rats, it would appear that, under adverse nutritional conditions puberty simply waits until the body has grown, however slowly, to approximately its normal puberal size or to its genetically determined maturity.

In the light of the secular trend in menarche and puberal growth spurt and the advances in nutrition and generally improved environmental conditions, it is not surprising, then, that there has also been a marked increase in body size at all age levels. Figure 37 illustrates this secular trend in heights and weights of Swedish school children with a separate recording of the age ranges of 7 to 14 years from the elementary schools and of 10 to 18 from the secondary schools. It also indicates that differences between these

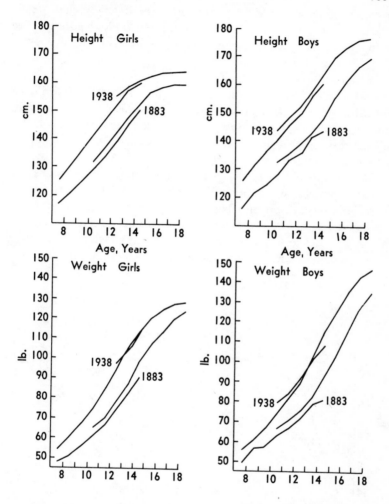

Figure 37. Secular trend in growth in height and weight. Height (above) and weight (below) of Swedish girls and boys measured in 1883 and 1938/39. Elementary schools age 7 to 14, secondary schools 10 to 18. (From J. M. Tanner, **Growth at Adolescence.** Oxford, Eng.: Blackwell Scientific Publications. By permission of the publisher.)

two school populations were greater in both height and weight for both sexes in 1883 than in 1938. This is undoubtedly a reflection of greater socio-economic differences between the groups in 1883.

A similar secular trend of increased body size and weight in American children has been noted over a forty year period. Figure 38 illustrates the changes from 1892 to the 1930's for girls, while similar results for boys indicate a difference in height of 2.3 inches at 11 years and 3.3 inches at 16 years favoring the 1930 grouping (Jones and Jones, 1957).

As with the advent of the menarche, regional variations are also noted in growth in height and weight. Although such variations may be expected on the basis of regional differences in socio-economic status, it appears that, in some instances, these differences are so great as to overcome the socio-economic factors. The differences in height and weight for girls in Kansas, California, and

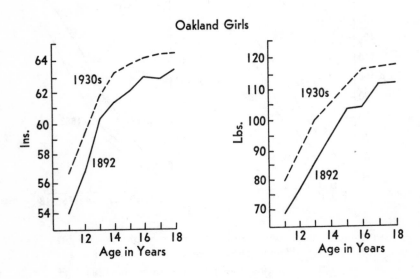

Figure 38.   A secular trend as shown in growth curves for girls. (From H. E. Jones and M. C. Jones, **Adolescence.** Berkeley: University Extension, University of California, 1957. By permission of the publisher.)

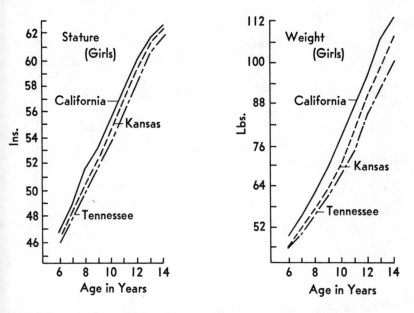

Figure 39.   Growth in height and weight: regional com-
               parisons. (From H. E. Jones and M. C. Jones,
               Adolescence. Berkeley: University Extension,
               University of California, 1957. By permission
               of the publisher.)

Tennessee illustrated in Figure 39 are such an example. Here the
lower of two social groups in California was on the average taller
and heavier at each age than the higher social group in Tennessee
(Jones and Jones, 1957).

   A similar comparison of boys measured at the University of Iowa
Child Welfare Station with boys in the Oakland Growth Study
indicates that the California boys achieved greater growth in height
even though the social status of the Iowa boy's parents was somewhat superior (Jones and Jones, 1957). Figure 40 gives the growth
curves of these two groups and also the amount of gain in height.
It clearly indicates that the growth of the Iowa and California boys
was similar in childhood but the California group grew more

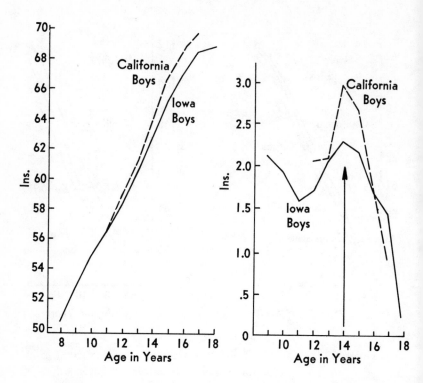

Figure 40.   Growth in height: Iowa and California boys.
                 (From H. E. Jones and M. C. Jones, **Adoles-
                 cence.** Berkeley: University Extension, Univer-
                 sity of California, 1957. By permission of the
                 publisher.)

rapidly during adolescence. This more rapid growth spurt on the
part of the California boys at puberty may be, in part, an explanation of their greater height in subsequent years.

SEASONAL VARIATIONS IN GROWTH

Well-defined seasonal variations have been found to exist in the
rate of growth in both height and weight at all age levels, includ-

ing adolescence, with growth in weight being fastest in the autumn and growth in height fastest in spring. Figure 41 shows the seasonal variations in the rate of weight gain of children in the northern hemisphere. October, November, and December are the months of greatest increase, with this weight increment sometimes being five or six times the amount of gain during the minimal increment months of April, May, and June. In general, over a six-month period, two-thirds of the annual weight gain is made between September and the end of February and the remaining one-third between the months of March and the end of August. These seasonal variations are imposed upon the general growth curve and, during periods of low rate of growth, it is possible for a small per-

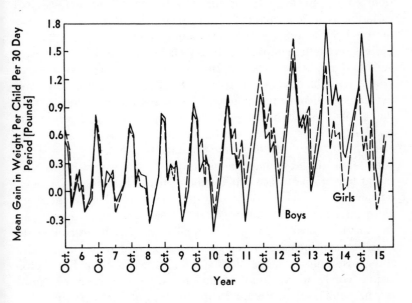

Figure 41.   Seasonal variation in weight gain, as observed in yearly age groups of elementary school children, Hagerstown, Md. (From C. E. Palmer, "Seasonal Variations of Average Growth in Weight of Elementary School Children." **Pbl. Hlth. Rep., Wash.,** 48:211-233, 1933.)

centage of children to actually lose weight during the spring months (Palmer, 1933). Even upon termination of the growth period such seasonal variation exists with adults showing weight gains averaging about one pound in the fall and loss of the corresponding amount in the spring (Kemsley, 1953).

The maximum height gains in childhood and adolescence are made at the same time minimal increases are recorded in weight. The majority of data indicate that 55 to 57 percent of the annual gain in height is made between the beginning of April and the end of September, with the average rate of gain during the months of April, May, and June being 2 to 2½ times that during the months of October, November, and December. More new ossification centers appear in the spring than in the fall, so that seasonal variation in skeletal maturity tends to coincide with seasonal variations in height gain (Reynolds and Sontag, 1944).

Since strength is more highly correlated with weight than with height, it might be expected that seasonal variations in strength should resemble the weight pattern. Such is not the case, however, for seasonal increments in strength and height gains coincide, with the greatest gains in strength being made in April while the smallest gains or, in the case of the girls, the greatest losses, are made in October. Although the seasonal variations are similar in both sexes, the absolute increments for boys are greater, as they would have to be to account for their greater increase in strength, but, even with the lesser increments, the seasonal differences are more marked in girls (Jones, 1949). The apparent seasonal discrepancy between weight and strength gains may be attributed to a lag between increases in muscular mass, as represented by weight, and gains in muscular functioning as indicated in strength measurements. Furthermore, total weight includes an element of "dead weight" which is uncorrelated with strength and it is possible that this "dead weight" gain is minimal during periods of rapid gain in height.

CHANGES IN BODY PROPORTIONS

The physical changes associated with sexual maturation of the individual reach their peak during the period of adolescence. One

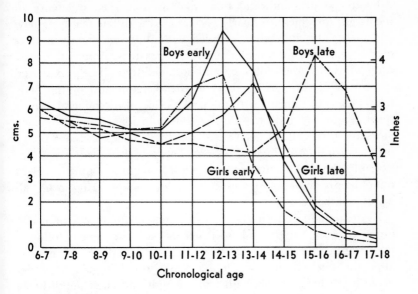

Figure 42.   Average yearly increments of growth in standing height for early- as compared to late-maturing boys and girls (late and early categories determined by age of maximum growth). (From J. E. Horrocks, "The Adolescent." In L. Carmichael (Ed.), **Manual of Child Psychology.** New York: John Wiley & Sons, Inc., 1954. By permission of the publisher.)

of the earliest manifestations of such maturation is the puberal growth spurt which, as with previously mentioned indices of maturation, appears first in female children. In girls, this growth spurt lasts from about 11 to 13½ years of age during which time the peak height gain averages 3¼ inches per year while in boys the growth spurt begins about 2 years later, from 13 to 15½ years, and has a peak gain in height growth of about 4 inches per year. Figure 42, based on data by Shuttleworth (1939), illustrates this earlier growth spurt in girls and points up the fact that it is of a lesser magnitude for girls than for boys.

Figure 42 also indicates that there is a marked difference in the height increments for early as compared with late maturing boys and girls. This difference, coupled with differential growth rates of the various segments of the body, tends to sculpture the body configuration of the adolescent and postadolescent. The peak period of growth of the various parts of the skeleton and of the body tissues tends to coincide with the peak period of the puberal growth spurt. Figure 43 indicates this general coincidence in three body measures with gain in height and weight in males and also points up the variations in rates of increase between these body areas. For example, the slight spurt in hand length prior to the spurt in height undoubtedly accounts for the early adolescent appearing to be "all hands and feet".

Reynolds and Schoen (1947), using longitudinal data of males, found that leg length tends to reach its peak first and is followed four months later by hip width and chest breadth. A few months after the peak of hip width and chest breadth gain, shoulder breadth reaches its peak, with trunk length and chest depth being the last of the skeletal measurements to achieve their peak gain. Since approximately one year separates the peaks of leg length and trunk length gains, the peak gain in stature consequently lies between the two. However, as more of the gain in height can be attributed to increases in trunk length than to leg length during this time, the peak in stature gain tends to be closer to the peak of trunk length gain.

A quick glance at Figure 42 would seem to indicate that early maturing girls and boys grow taller than the late maturers on the basis of a lesser gain of the latter in peak height increments. However, such is not the case, since the late maturers grow over a longer period of time and, although they may be shorter during the early part of the adolescent period, they tend to be as tall or taller during adulthood. Measurement of 188 cadet officers at the Royal Military Academy in Sandhurst by Tanner (1955) revealed that there was a strict relationship between adult height and maturity grouping with the latest maturers being the tallest.

A study of the relationship between weight and menarche indicates that early maturers are consistently heavier and late maturers consistently lighter between the ages of 6 to 18 years (Richey, 1937).

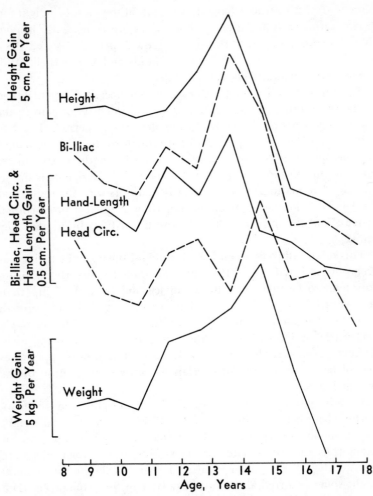

Figure 43.   Adolescent spurts in various body measure-
              ments. The curves are arranged one beneath
              the other without regard to zero on the
              vertical scale. Average figures for 3 mono-
              vular triplets, each measured at each age.
              (From J. M. Tanner, **Growth at Adolescence.**
              Oxford, Eng.: Blackwell Scientific Publica-
              tions, 1955. By permission of the publisher.)

Numerous investigations have shown that on the basis of weight-for-height ratios early maturers of both sexes are consistently heavier than late maturers over the entire growth period (Pryor, 1936; Shuttleworth, 1939; Bayley, 1943; Reynolds and Wines, 1948; Wilson and Sutherland, 1950; Tanner, 1955).

The linearity of late maturers can, in some measure, be attributed to the variations in sequence, duration, and intensity of gain in the various segments of the body during the growth period. The late maturers have a longer period of leg growth so that the leg length becomes proportionately greater than trunk length. Furthermore, the gain during the peak periods for the various segments is not as great for late maturers as it is for early maturers with the result that the later developing segments do not have as great a proportional increase and the individual has a more linear body build (See Figure 42).

This relationship between body build and timing of maturing has been observed by Bayley (1943) also. She noted that early maturing boys tend to be relatively shorter of leg and broader of hip than late maturing boys. Conversely, late maturing girls have a growth spurt resembling that of boys with these girls having relatively longer legs and broader shoulders than the early maturing girls. However, even here the general body configuration only approaches that of boys and would not overlap the body configuration of the average boy.

A study of the growth curves of 26 ectomorphic and 28 mesomorphic boys between the ages of 2 to 17 years indicates that weight growth for mesomorphs is similar to that of early maturers and for ectomorphs to that of late maturers. Moreover, ectomorphs were consistently taller at all ages after 4 years. Peaks in the puberal height spurt occurred about one year later in the ectomorphs (Dupertuis and Michael, 1953). Similarly, a significantly greater percentage of endomesomorphic boys are advanced than retarded in skeletal maturity (Clarke, Irving and Heath, 1961) while slow skeletal maturers are predominantly ectomorphic (Acheson and Dupertuis, 1957).

Studies of the relationship between somatotype and the menarche by Barker and Stone (1936), who used the Kretschmerian body

typing, revealed that pyknic (obese) women have their first menstruation approximately 8 months earlier than leptosomic (thin)
women. Similarly, girls with a slender body build tend to menstru-
ate later than girls with a broad build (Pryor, 1936).

Sex differences in body build become noteworthy after puberty.
In general, the chief skeletal differences between adult men and
women are in overall size and in greater shoulder width and limb
length in men and broader hips in women. The relatively longer
arm of the male when the sexes are equated for size is due mainly
to a sex difference in the development of the forearm (Dupertuis

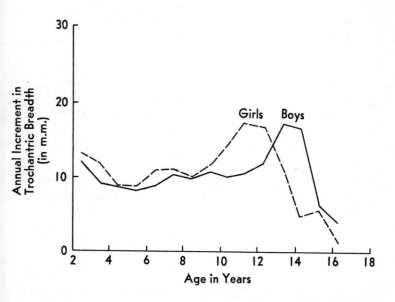

Figure 44.   Annual increments in trochantric (hip) breadth.
              (Adapted from data by K. Simmons, "The
              Brush Foundation Study of Child Growth and
              Development. II. Physical Growth and De-
              velopment." **Monogr. Soc. Res. Child De-
              velpm.**, 9(1):1-87, 1944.)

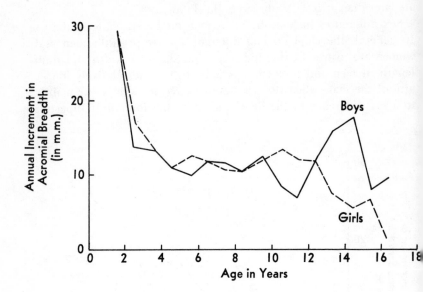

Figure 45.   Annual increments in acromial (shoulder)
                  breadth. (Adapted from data by K. Simmons,
                  "The Brush Foundation Study of Child Growth
                  and Development. II. Physical Growth and
                  Development." **Monogr. Soc. Res. Child De-**
                  velpm., 9(1):1-87, 1944.)

and Hadden, 1951). This difference is already established at 2 years
and is increased during the period from 2 years to adolescence by
the continuously greater relative growth rate of the forearm to the
upper arm in boys (Maresh, 1943). The data of Meredith and Boynton (1937) indicate that this sex difference also extends to the circumference of the forearm as well as the length of the segment.

Variations between the sexes in hip and shoulder width may be
attributed to differential sex hormone secretions. Figure 44 indicates
that the rate of gain in hip width tends to be the same for both

sexes but continues slightly longer for girls so that they will, on this basis alone, have slightly larger relative hip widths than boys. In shoulder width, however, girls have a relatively low gain in comparison with the marked gain for boys (Figure 45). It is this latter low segmental growth that accounts for the relatively larger hipped, narrower shouldered configuration of women (Simmons, 1944) .

PHYSIOLOGICAL CHANGES

Adolescence is marked by a number of physiological changes, other than those directly associated with puberty, which affect the physical performance of the sexes. One of these changes involves the basal heart rate which has been falling gradually and equally for both sexes since birth. Although this decrease continues for both sexes during adolescence, it is much more marked in males than in females (Figure 46) after the age of 12 years (Iliff and Lee, 1952), until in adulthood the resting heart rate of women is 10 percent greater than in men (Boas and Goldschmidt, 1932).

Associated with changes in heart rate are changes in basal body temperature. Tanner (1951) points out that, in healthy persons, heart rate is closely related to body temperature in that for every degree F that an individual's resting oral temperature lies above the average, the heart rate also lies 11 beats per minute above the average. Therefore, it is not surprising that the basal body temperature continues to drop from birth by an equal amount in both sexes until approximately 12 years when the decline levels off in girls but continues in boys (Iliff and Lee, 1952). The sex difference of about one-half degree in body temperature that results persists into adult life (Cullumbine, 1949).

Systolic blood pressure has been found to rise steadily during childhood with a much more rapid increase during adolescence until adult values are reached (Richey, 1931; Downing, 1947). As with other measures, the changes occur first in girls but the boys' adolescent rise, when it appears, is greater than the girls' increase, with the resultant difference accounting for the higher resting systolic pressure in young adult males (Figure 47).

Adolescence brings only a very slight change in the diastolic blood pressure with no statistically significant differences between

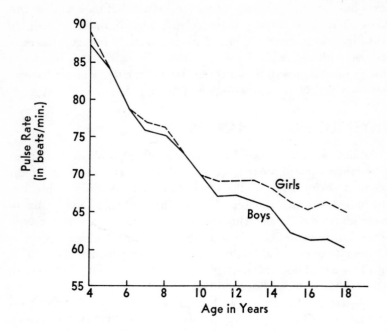

Figure 46.   Curves of average basal heart rates for boys
                   and girls. (Adapted from data by A. Iliff and
                   V. A. Lee, "Pulse Rate, Respiratory Rate,
                   and Body Temperature of Children Between
                   Two Months and Eighteen Years of Age."
                   Child Develpm., 23:237-245, 1952.)

the sexes (Shock, 1944). Therefore, the changes in pulse pressure parallel those in systolic blood pressure (Figure 48). It has been suggested that the greater increase in heart size in males during adolescence results in the establishment of a greater basal stroke volume which accounts for the increased pulse pressure and systolic blood pressure (Nylin, 1935).

An additional cause for the higher systolic blood pressure in males may be their increased blood volume (Tanner, 1955). Although there is no sex difference with respect to blood volume before puberty in relation to the height or weight of the individual, a

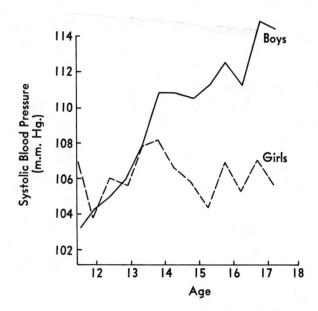

Figure 47.   Curves of average systolic blood pressure of
boys and girls. (From N. W. Shock, "Basal
Blood Pressure and Pulse Rate in Adolescents."
Amer. J. Dis. Child., 68:16-22, 1944. By permission of the author and publisher.)

greater increase in boys has been noted during adolescence which
results in a higher male adult value (Sjöstrand, 1953). This higher
blood volume in the young male adult also reflects a large increase
in red blood cells for boys during adolescence.

Mugrage and Andresen (1936, 1938) report a greater rise in the
number of red blood corpuscles in boys and a consequent increase
in the hemoglobin of the blood in comparison with girls (Figures 49
and 50). These increases are accomplished with little or no changes
in mean corpuscular volume, mean corpuscular hemoglobin, or
mean corpuscular hemoglobin concentration (Mugrage and Andresen, 1936, 1938; Berry et al., 1952). Girls do not exhibit this increase

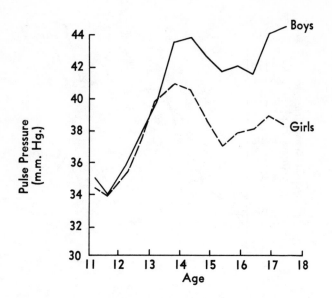

Figure 48.   Curves of average pulse pressures of boys and
girls. (From N. W. Shock, "Basal Blood Pres-
sure and Pulse Rate in Adolescents." **Amer.
J. Dis. Child.,** 68:16-22, 1944. By permission
of the author and publisher.)

in red blood cells and consequent increase in hemoglobin during
adolescence nor do well-trained women athletes achieve sufficient increases in both areas to eliminate this sex difference (Marloff, 1949).

An increase in red blood cells and in hemoglobin volume requires
a complementary increase in available oxygen for its effective use
in the body. During adolescence, basal respiratory rate shows no sex
difference nor any variation in the consistent fall noted from birth
(Iliff and Lee, 1952). However, there are changes in the respiratory
volume, vital capacity, and maximum breathing capacity. The resting respiratory volume, both on a per minute and per breath basis,
increases considerably in boys but very little in girls (Shock, 1946).

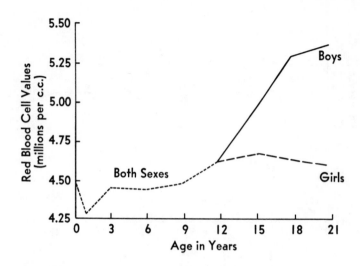

Figure 49.   Mean red blood cell values in boys and girls.
               (From data by E. R. Mugrage and M. I.
               Andresen, "Values for Red Blood Cells of
               Average Infants and Children." **Amer. J. Dis.
               Child.,** 51:775-791, 1936. E. R. Mugrage and
               M. I. Andresen, "Red Blood Cell Values in
               Adolescence." **Amer. J. Dis. Child.,** 56:997-
               1003, 1938. By permission of the authors and
               publisher.)

Similarly, the maximum breathing capacity, which is the volume
breathed during a 15 second period in which the subject breathes as
deeply and rapidly as possible, and the vital capacity, namely, the
maximal expiration following a maximal inspiration, have been
found to show a considerable adolescent increase for boys but not
for girls (Figures 51 and 52). The increases in boys are larger than
can be accounted for simply by the increase in body size, with boys
having a greater vital capacity for the same body surface area than

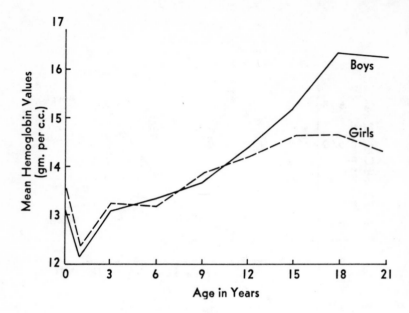

Figure 50. Mean hemoglobin values in boys and girls. (From data by E. R. Mugrage and M. I. Andresen, "Values for Red Blood Cells of Average Infants and Children." **Amer. J. Dis. Child.**, 51:775-791, 1936. E. R. Mugrage and M. I. Andresen, "Red Blood Cell Values in Adolescence." **Amer. J. Dis. Child.**, 56:997-1003, 1938. By permission of the authors and publisher.)

girls after puberty (Tanner, 1955). It is believed that this phenomenon reflects a greater inside growth in the lungs of boys corresponding to the outside increases in shoulder and chest width (Morse et al., 1952).

Additional respiratory changes in both sexes involve a decrease in the percentage of oxygen and an increase in the amount of carbon dioxide in the expired air, with these changes occurring to a greater extent in boys than in girls at puberty (Shock and Soley, 1939). Alveolar carbon dioxide tension increases in boys but not in girls,

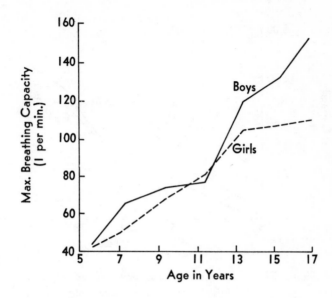

Figure 51.   Curves of average maximum breathing capacity in boys and girls. (From data by B. G.
Ferris, J. L. Whittenberger and J. R. Gallagher, "Maximum Breathing Capacity and
Vital Capacity of Male Children and Adolescents." **Pediatrics,** 9:659-670, 1952. B. G.
Ferris and C. W. Smith, "Maximum Breathing
Capacity and Vital Capacity in Female Children and Adolescents." **Pediatrics,** 12:341-
352, 1953. By permission of the authors and
publisher.)

so that a sex difference appears after the age of 13 years (Shock,
1941). These changes, together with the observation by Robinson
(1938) that the alkali reserve of boys rises at puberty, result in the
male's blood being able to absorb greater quantities of lactic acid
and other muscular metabolites during muscular exercise than can
a woman's blood without a change in the Ph of the blood. Such an
adjustment would seem to be a necessity due to the relatively greater

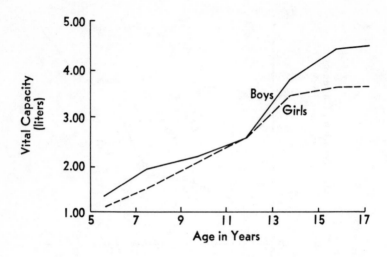

Figure 52.   Curves of average vital capacity in boys and
girls. (From data by B. G. Ferris, J. L. Whittenberger and J. R. Gallagher, "Maximum
Breathing Capacity and Vital Capacity of
Male Children and Adolescents." **Pediatrics,**
9:659-670, 1952. B. G. Ferris and C. W.
Smith, "Maximum Breathing Capacity and
Vital Capacity in Female Children and Adolescents." **Pediatrics,** 12:341-352, 1953. By
permission of the authors and publisher.)

development of muscular bulk in males during the adolescent
growth spurt.

The increase in respiratory volume and decrease in the percentage of oxygen in expired air of boys reflects the increased oxygen
consumption that has been noted in males at puberty (Garn and
Clark, 1953). This increase is closely associated with changes in
basal metabolism rate during adolescence. The basal metabolic rate,
which is the amount of heat produced per square meter of body
surface under resting conditions, falls continuously from birth to
old age. However, the data of Lewis et al, (1943) indicate that the

basal metabolic rate is consistently higher in boys than for girls and that this difference becomes greater during the period of adolescence when the decline in rate for boys is arrested to a greater extent than it is in girls (Figures 53 and 54). This relative increase, or slowing down of the declining rate, coincides with the adolescent growth spurt and is indicative of the extra heat production that would appear to be inseparable from the building of new tissue although there may also be some contributions from the hormonal effects of the thyroid or of androgens in the male.

The greater metabolic rate and oxygen consumption relative to surface area of boys in comparison with girls at all age levels has

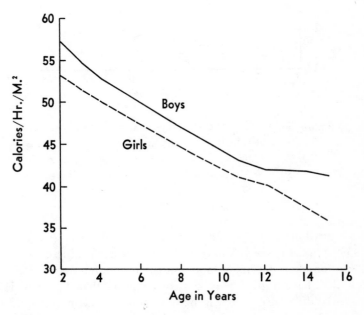

Figure 53.   Curves of average basal metabolic rate in boys and girls. (Adapted from data by R. C. Lewis, A. M. Duval and A. Iliff, "Standards for the Basal Metabolism of Children from 2 to 15 Years of Age, Inclusive." **J. Pediat.,** 23:1-18, 1943.)

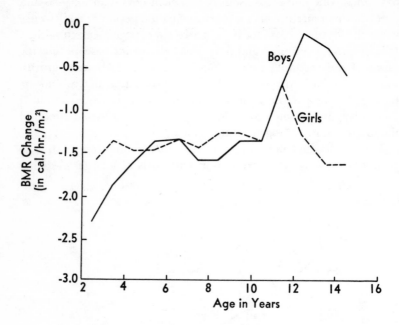

Figure 54.   Curves of average change in basal metabolic
rate in boys and girls. (Adapted from data
by R. C. Lewis, A. M. Duval and A. Iliff,
"Standards for the Basal Metabolism of Children from 2 to 15 Years of Age, Inclusive."
J. Pediat., 23:1-18, 1943.)

been attributed to the greater mesomorphy of boys (Garn et al.,
1953). Muscle tissue is known to have a greater resting oxygen consumption than fat tissue and muscular children have also been
found to have a greater oxygen consumption than fat ones. However, the differences noted in body size and muscle mass would not
seem to be great enough to account for the amount of sex difference,
nor of the increase in the sex difference, during adolescence. A
comparison of boys and girls with the same muscular bulk as measured by x-rays of the calf revealed that boys had a higher oxygen
consumption per kilogram of body weight. A difference has also

been found to exist between the strength of males and females with the same muscular bulk (Rarick and Thompson, 1956; Morris, 1948). It is possible that male hormone secretions account for such differences and their heightened production during adolescence and adulthood increases sex differences in muscular metabolism.

CHANGES IN BODY TISSUES

Marked proportional changes occur in the bone, muscle, and fat tissues at adolescence. As may be expected, gains in bone and muscle parallel increments in height and weight. Figure 55, based upon the longitudinal data collected on three monovular triplets (Reynolds and Schoen, 1947), gives a very clear picture of the spurt in bone and muscle. It also indicates the inverse relationship between these two measures and fat deposition during the peak growth period. While this decrement in fat gain is very marked in boys, it has a much lesser magnitude in girls (Figure 24). Here fat gains are also consistently higher at all ages. In general, girls appear to have an equally intense gain in bone and muscle growth as boys but do not have the same duration of gain nor as pronounced a reduction in fat gain during adolescence.

A study by Reynolds (1944) of 48 girls and 30 boys between the ages of 7½ and 12½ years points up the differences in bone, muscle, and fat development for early and late maturers. The data indicate that early maturing girls are significantly larger than late maturers in the following measures: total calf breadth, 8½ through 12½ years; breadth of fat, all ages; breadth of muscle, 10½ through 12 years; and breadth of bone, 8½ through 12½ years. During the period from 7½ to 12½ years, early maturing girls show a mean increase in total calf breadth of 26.5 mm. while the late maturing increase only 11.9 mm. The boys' data indicate early maturers are larger than the late maturers in mean calf breadth and in fat, muscle, and bone from 9½ through 12½ years, although the differences are not as great as in girls. The main differential in boys appears to be the faster rate of growth in fat breadth in late maturers, although early maturing boys are, as are early maturing girls, consistently larger in fat breadth at every age.

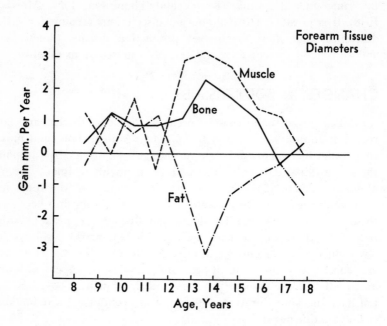

Figure 55.   Adolescent spurt in bone, muscle and subcutaneous fat diameters of the forearm, taken
at right angles to long axis of limb one-third
of way up forearm from distal end of radial
diaphysis, by X-ray. Average of 3 monovular
male triplets. (From J. M. Tanner, **Growth
at Adolescence.** Oxford, Eng.: Blackwell Scientific Publications, 1955. By permission of
the publisher.)

STRENGTH INCREMENTS

The marked physiological and structural changes of the adolescent growth spurt are reflected in large increments and sex differences in strength development. Jones (1949) has reported the results
from a longitudinal study of static muscular strength development
undertaken at the University of California Institute of Child Wel-

fare with approximately 90 subjects of each sex from 11 through
17½ years of age. Development of strength in hand grip, arm pull,
and arm thrust is nearly the same for both boys and girls until after
13 years when the boys increase in strength much more rapidly than
the girls. A comparison of changes relative to initial status indicates
the total amount of change in gripping strength for boys is almost
twice as great as for girls (See Figures 57 and 58), while for pulling
and thrusting strength the total amount of change is approximately
four times as great.

Previously reported studies of strength during childhood indicated the great variability of strength within the sexes, so that there
is considerable overlapping of the strength measures of stronger girls
with those of boys. Figure 56 shows that such overlapping is greatly
reduced after the adolescent growth spurt, with no girls exceeding
the average strength of the boys in the measures tested by Jones
(1949). There is, however, still a great deal of variability in strength
within the sexes and the strongest girls may still equal or slightly
surpass the weakest boys in strength.

Maturity indices have a decided relationship to strength development. When classified as early, average, and late maturers according
to age at menarche, the growth curves in strength of the late maturing girls lag behind the average at all ages. The early maturers
exhibit a tendency toward more rapid growth in strength from 11
to 13 years but their growth is retarded relatively soon thereafter
and they reach a terminal position below the group mean (Jones,
1949). Figure 57, illustrating the growth curve of right hand grip
strength, shows the tendency for both early and late maturers to be
weaker than average maturing girls after 13½ years of age.

The differences in strength growth curves of early, average, and
late maturing boys, assessed on the basis of skeletal age, are illustrated in Figure 58. The early maturers exhibit a growth curve that
is not far from linear, with acceleration usually falling between 12
and 13½ years and a tendency to level off after the 16th or 17th
year. The late maturing boys, on the other hand, reveal two phases
of growth, namely, a slow increase in each function followed by an
acceleration at 14 years or later. There is also a marked relationship
between strength and skeletal maturity, in that the early maturing
boys are above the group mean in strength from ages 13 through 16

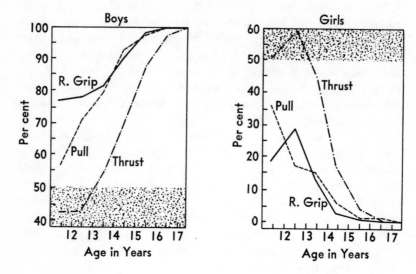

Figure 56. Percentage of boys and girls surpassing the mean of the opposite sex in various strength measures. (From H. E. Jones, **Motor Performance and Growth.** Berkeley: University of California Press, 1949. By permission of the publisher.)

while the late maturers tend to fall below the norm at these ages. Within minor variation, each individual maintains approximately his same position relative to his age mates. Those boys who were superior in strength at the beginning of the Oakland Growth Study remained superior at its termination while those who were in the lower percentile also tended to remain in about the same relative position. Since early maturity has also been associated with mesomorphy and late maturity with ectomorphy, it is not surprising that strength is moderately related to mesomorphy and slightly negatively related to ectomorphy (Jones, 1949).

However, the low correlations that have been obtained between either height or weight and strength suggest that factors other than gross body size are influential in determining strength in adoles-

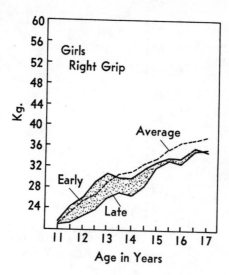

Figure 57.   Growth curves (right grip) for early-, average, and late-maturing girls, classified on the basis of age at menarche. (From H. E. Jones, **Motor Performance and Growth.** Berkeley: University of California Press, 1949. By permission of the publisher.)

cence (Jones, 1949). Additional longitudinal data indicate that the peak in strength spurt in boys occurs about 1½ years after the peak height increases and about 1 year after the peak weight gains (Dimock, 1935; Stolz and Stolz, 1951). Although there are no clear cut data available on the growth of muscles alone, it has been suggested that the peak gain of muscular growth coincides with, or even precedes, the peak weight gain (Tanner, 1955). Such discrepancy in peak gains seems to indicate that muscles grow first in size and later in strength.

Data on androgen excretion approximates the growth in strength for it continues to rise for a year or more after growth in height has practically ceased (Tanner, 1955). A close association may be made between strength and male hormonal secretions on the basis

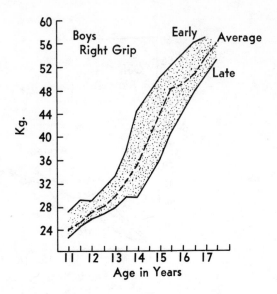

of studies by Simonson et al. (1941) which show an increase in the
muscular strength of eunuchs and castrates upon injection of methyl
testosterone and of Burke et al. (1953) showing a decline in grip
strength after the age of 30 years which generally resembles the decline in 17-ketosteroid output in males. In general, then, there is
a period of about one year between achievement of full body size
and the development of full muscular power in the male which
may be attributed to the effects of the male hormones upon the
proteins and enzymes of the muscle fibers.

CHANGES IN MOTOR PERFORMANCE

As may be expected, changes in motor performance tend to
parallel the changes in body size, strength, and physiological func-

tioning at puberty. Sex differences in basic motor skill performances become increasingly marked, with boys showing continued improvement whereas performance increments for girls are negligible or, in some instances, decline after menarche. Figures 25 and 62 illustrate these changes in running; Figures 27 and 63 in the standing broad jump; and Figures 28 and 64 in the throw for distance. In the study cited, girls reached their maximum in running at 13 years and showed little change in distance throwing and jumping after this age (Espenschade, 1960). More recent cross-sectional studies which coincide with an emphasis on physical fitness suggest a somewhat different trend. In California, for example, slight improvement in running and jumping was noted for girls from 13 to 16 years. Failure of girls to improve after puberty in physical performance is apparently strongly influenced by the cultural milieu.

When performances are related to skeletal or menarcheal age in girls, it must be recognized that each of these correlated substantially with chronological age. When motor performance of girls is graphed in relation to skeletal maturity (Figures 59 and 60), motor performance has either leveled off, as in the dash, or has been declining steadily, as in the distance throw, with increased skeletal maturity. Treatment of these same data on the basis of age of deviation from menarche reveals similar results. However, in this instance, there were very few cases more than .5 years before the menarche. In general, motor performance of girls in basic skills tends to level off shortly before the achievement of biological maturity, which is reached approximately 3 years prior to skeletal maturity (Espenschade, 1940).

Conversely, boys continue to improve in motor performance with increasing skeletal maturity (Figures 59 and 60). However, the skeletal rating range in Figures 59 and 60 does not include the rating of 37, which signifies skeletal maturity in boys, and it is possible that the graphed relationship may, to some extent, be a function of the interrelationships between skeletal maturity and other physical maturity measures such as chronological age, height, and weight (Espenschade, 1940). Partial correlation techniques have produced results indicating that skeletal age accounts for less than 9 percent of the variance in motor performance (Rarick and Oyster, 1964).

Variation in the rate of skeletal development does, however, bear some relationship to motor performance in boys as was noted in the

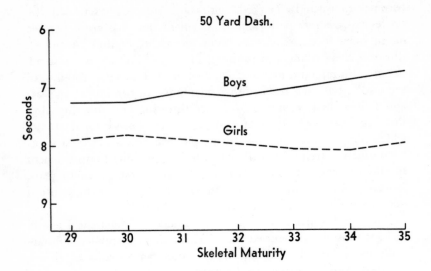

Figure 59.   Curves of skeletal maturity and performance
in the 50 yard dash for boys and girls. (From
Anna S. Espenschade, "Motor Performance
in Adolescence Including the Study of Relationships with Measures of Physical Growth
and Maturity." **Monogr. Soc. Res. Child Develpm.,** 5(1):1-126, 1940. By permission of the
publisher.)

preceding chapter. When boys at 9, 12, and 15 years from the Medford, Oregon, Boys' Growth Project were categorized into retarded,
normal, and advanced maturers, the advanced maturers had higher
performance means in strength measures and in the standing broad
jump than retarded maturers. In general, it was found that the highest and most significant differences between maturity groupings were
obtained at 15 years with those at 12 and 9 years being of decreasing order with chronological age. Furthermore, a comparison of the
chronological ages within similar maturity groupings indicated that
the chronologically older boys were taller and stronger (Clarke and
Harrison, 1962).

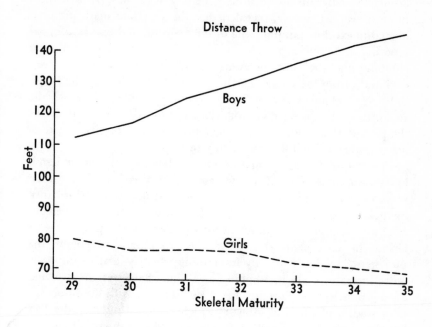

Figure 60. Curves of skeletal maturity and performance
in the distance throw for boys and girls.
(From Anna S. Espenschade, "Motor Performance in Adolescence Including the Study
of Relationships with Measures of Physical
Growth and Maturity." **Monogr. Soc. Res.
Child Develpm.,** 5(1):1-126, 1940. By permission of the publisher.)

Studies of the relationship between motor performance and
pubescence reveal a similar slight relationship for boys and little
relationship for girls. The few records that are available for girls do
not present a parallel picture with previously reported strength development where the average maturers eventually exceeded both the
early and late developers (Jones, 1949). Atkinson (1925) grouped
9000 Philadelphia high school girls on the basis of deviation from
menarche and found no marked differences in comparison with

arrangement by chronological age. A study of the best performances in each event, however, revealed that the very late maturing girls tended to excel in jumping, the distance throw, and basketball goal shooting while the early maturing girls were more proficient in rope climbing and the running events. Similarly, correlations between deviations from the menarche and performance events in the longitudinal Oakland Growth Study were negligible (Espenschade, 1940). It would appear then, that the advent of the menarche marks the peak of steady increase in motor performances of girls but does not necessarily signal the end of all growth.

The rate of biological maturation for boys, on the other hand, has shown some relationship to motor performance. Low correlations ranging from .06 to .37 were obtained between performance in the various events in the Oakland Growth study and pubescent zone, or stage, but some differences were noted in the percentage of change in performance in the various groupings. In general, the pubescent boy gains steadily in running whereas relative improvement increases early in jumping and somewhat later in throwing during pubescence (Espenschade, 1940). These results are in accord with studies of physical growth sequence indicating that the legs lengthen and the hips widen prior to shoulder girdle development.

When a combined motor performance score for five track events, including runs, jumps, and the shot put, was graphed against McCloy's Classification Index scores for each of three pubescent groupings, the pre- and postpubescent boys improved steadily in each classification grouping while pubescent boys of all classes scored approximately the same number of motor performance points. The prepubescent boys tended to be slightly better in performance than the pubescents at the higher classification index ranges for these groups but the rate of gain and the actual motor performance scores were greater for the postpubescents at all overlapping indices (Nevers, 1948).

Similarly, the participants in the 1955 Little League World Series, who ranged in age from 10 to 12 years, were found to be mainly pubescent and postpubescent (Hale, 1956). At 13 and 16 years, boys in the Medford, Oregon Boys' Growth Study who were advanced in pubescent development had higher mean scores on various motor ability tests with the most effective differentiation by pubescent assessment occurring at 13 years. As with skeletal age, differences between various pubescent groupings are also partially conditioned by chronological age. Boys who are older chronologically, but with the same pubescent rating, generally have significantly higher mean performance scores (Clarke and Degutis, 1962).

In relation to his peers, therefore, the early maturing boy has decided advantages in terms of body size and build, strength, and possibly physiological functioning which allow him to excel in physical performance during adolescence.

MOTOR COORDINATION AND BALANCE

Although the total scores on the Brace test indicate that there is a steady increase with chronological age for boys, whereas girls show no improvement after 14 years (Figure 29), these total scores are a composite of 20 items, each of which is scored on a pass or fail basis. An analysis of performance in the individual items reveals growth patterns which are masked in the total score. In several of the items sex differences are not as great as the total scores would imply, while in others the differences are greater. For example, the stunt which requires the subject to "fold arms across the chest, cross the feet and sit down crosslegged, then stand again without unfolding the arms and moving the feet from the floor" shows the least amount of sex difference and the least amount of variation over the entire age range for both sexes. Events in which boys are especially superior are those agility items requiring rapid change of direction of the body or its parts such as jumping full turns with the position held at the finish and jumping through a loop made by grasping a foot in the opposite hand. These agility measures present a greater problem for older girls than for younger ones, but in stunts requiring control or static balance older girls are able to maintain their position (Espenschade, 1947).

It is possible that the decline in agility in girls after 14 years, whereas little change is shown in control, flexibility, and balance items, may be attributed to lack of interest rather than to actual decline in capacity. Longitudinal data from the Oakland Growth Study where the subjects had practice during the process of being tested every six months, indicates a slight increase for the total

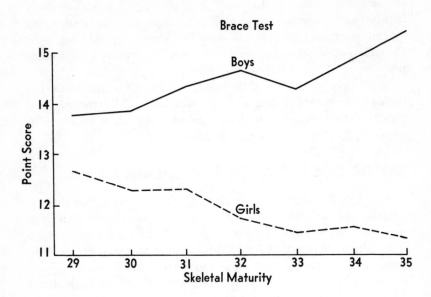

scores of the Brace test up to 16 years (Espenschade, 1940). However, when these same data are analyzed in terms of skeletal maturity (Figure 61), a decline is noted with increasing skeletal age.
This decline may reflect increased pubertal weight with its negative
effect on motor performance in girls as much as the changed interests and attitudes which accompany biological maturity.

Figure 61 also indicates that boys show increased performance
with skeletal age except for a slight decline between the skeletal
maturity ratings of 32 and 33. When these longitudinal data were
supplemented with additional cross-sectional data, little gain was

found in total test scores between 12½ and 14 years. An analysis of the items of the Brace test shows increased ability to perform in events of all the sub-categories, with amount of gain being greater after 14 years than before this age. Furthermore, gains are more rapid in agility than in control events. On the other hand, test items in which dynamic balance can be considered a factor show a marked adolescent lag and it is possible that these items play the largest role in the reduction of increases in the composite Brace score during the period from 12½ to 14 years (Espenschade, 1947).

Although higher mean scores are reported from 13 to 16 years for prepubescent boys, an analysis of the rate of gain over a two year period revealed a pattern of increase before puberty, a slackening in the rate of increase during the months around the time when a boy reaches pubescence, and further increase after puberty (Dimock, 1935). Reorganization of the Brace test data from the Oakland Growth Study with respect to pubescent status does not indicate any superiority of prepubescent boys, but does reveal each advancing state of maturity to be superior to that preceding except for the few cases which mark the earliest appearance of a stage or level (Espenschade et al., 1953). Such results indicate that motor coordination or ability, as measured by the Brace test, tends to increase less rapidly during the period of onset of puberty.

Various studies of dynamic balance during adolescence indicate a slackening in the rate of gain for both sexes. When measured on the walking board, this plateau in the rate of gain for girls appears from 12 through 14 years (Heath, 1949; Goetzinger, 1961). In some instances, steady improvement in performance on walking beams has been reported in boys up to 14 and 16 years (Heath, 1949; Goetzinger, 1961) while, in others, steady improvement was noted until 11 years with a subsequent decline in gain (Seashore, 1947) or greater variability (Wallon et al., 1958). Another study of boys aged 11½ to 16½ years shows consistent gains in beam walking with chronological age, although the rate of change is much less from 13 to 15 years than occurs earlier or later. Classification of the boys in this study into puberal groupings reveals similar results, with the pre-and postpubescent group curves both rising sharply while the intermediate pubescent groups show little gain (Espenschade et al., 1953).

Similarly, there is an apparent adverse effect during adolescence which occurs earlier in females than in males for balance as measured by the stabilometer. Conversely, however, this same group was superior in performance in a ladder-balancing task during adolescence in comparison with other periods (Bachman, 1961). This latter task may involve factors other than balance to a considerable extent, however. On the basis of a correlation coefficient of .62, it may be assumed that there is a substantial relationship between dynamic balance and ratings in physical ability of junior high school boys (Espenschade et al., 1953). Therefore, some indications should also be found of slight pubertal lag in other motor activities. Previously cited studies by Hale (1956), found only 17 perce it of Little League participants to be pubescent, while 37.5 and 45.5 percent were pre- and postpubescent respectively. Nevers (1948) reports pubescent boys as being poorer in achievement in track events at upper classification indices than were prepubescent boys. Both studies tend to suggest a slight adolescent lag in motor ability. It seems logical that rapid changes in physique, strength, and body proportions will require some readjustment of sensory-motor functioning, and it is possible the decreased rate of gain in balancing and motor ability noted by a number of investigators at puberty may be associated with such adjustments.

SECULAR TRENDS AND GEOGRAPHIC VARIATION IN MOTOR PERFORMANCE

The reported secular trend in increased height and weight at all ages implies that such a trend should also exist in motor performance. This is indeed the case and Figures 62 through 64 indicate increased performance for both boys and girls in running, jumping, and distance throwing over a period of 7 years. However, such a marked increase over so short a period of time does raise questions as to sampling of the respective groups and of possible influences of heightened interest in, and increased practice of, physical fitness test items. These figures are based upon the norms of the nationwide Youth Fitness Test surveys of 1958 and 1965.

A comparative study of motor performance of 13-year-old girls and 13½-year-old boys in the same region and with similar socio-

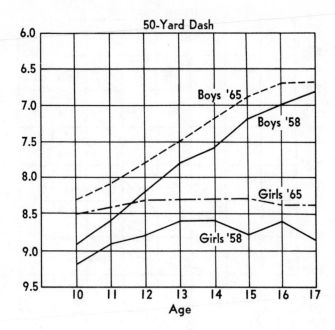

Figure 62.   Youth Fitness Test norms of 1958 and 1965
for the 50-yard dash. (From P. A. Hunsicker
and G. G. Reiff, "A Survey and Comparison
of Youth Fitness 1958-1965." **J. Health P. E.
Rec.,** 37:23-25, 1966. By permission of the
publisher.)

economic backgrounds does not show improved performance in all
test items over a 24-year period. Significant increases are noted in
height and weight for both sexes and conform with studies reporting
such increases over a much longer period of time. Such increases in
weight appear to be more advantageous for boys than girls, however. Boys register significant increases in performance in the distance throw, jump and reach, Brace test, grip, and pull whereas
girls improve significantly only in the jump and reach and pull.
The increase in height and weight appears to have had a detrimental effect on performance in the dash and standing broad jump

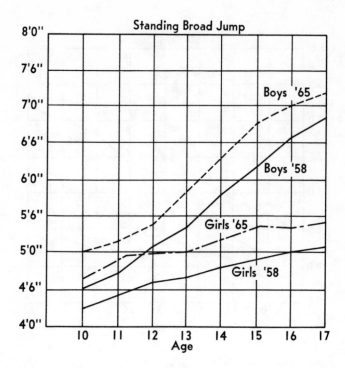

Figure 63.   Youth Fitness Test norms of 1958 and 1965
               for the standing broad jump. (From P. A.
               Hunsicker and G. G. Reiff, "A Survey and
               Comparison of Youth Fitness 1958-1965." **J.
               Health P. E. Rec.**, 37:23-25, 1966. By per-
               mission of the publisher.)

for both sexes, with significant decrements occurring in performance
levels. Girls also are significantly weaker in the push in 1958 in
comparison with their 1934 counterparts (Espenschade and Meleney,
1961). Norms for large groups of California children tested in 1960
are lower in dash and broad jump than those reported in California
children in the 1930's, also.

Previously reported studies generally tend to indicate a low, but
positive, correlation between height and weight and performance

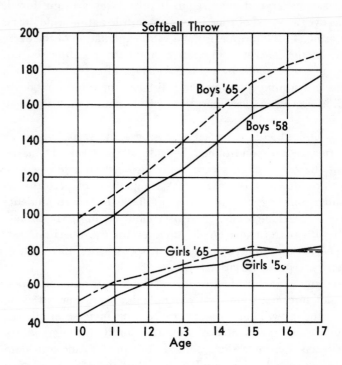

Softball Throw

Boys '65

Boys '58

Girls '65

Girls '5o

Age

Figure 64. Youth Fitness Test norms of 1958 and 1965 for the softball throw for distance. (From P. A. Hunsicker and G. G. Reiff, "A Survey and Comparison of Youth Fitness 1958-1965." **J. Health P. E. Rec.,** 37:23-25, 1966. By permission of the publisher.)

in the run and jump. Therefore, it is possible that the significant decrease registered by both sexes in the dash and standing broad jump is a reflection of decreased interest and opportunity for the achievement of individual optimal performance in these activities for the average boy and girl. Additional justification for such a conclusion is indicated by increased performance in these events by both sexes over the 7-year period between the nation-wide Physical Fitness Test surveys (Hunsicker and Reiff, 1966).

It may be argued that regional differences account for decrements over a period of time in one area while nation-wide norms are increasing. This, however, is not a valid explanation of the decreases noted in the 24-year comparative study since California, on the basis of scores made by over 200,000 children, had higher state norms in running, jumping, and distance throwing for both sexes at all age levels in 1958 than those of the nation-wide Physical Fitness Test.

It is undoubtedly a truism that geographic variations in motor performance are conditioned by cultural patterns. To a certain extent, however, basic motor skills also reflect noted geographic variations in onset of puberty. A comparison of performance in running, jumping, and throwing of 19,000 Bulgarian students between the ages of 8 and 20 years conducted in 1951 (Mangarov, 1964) with performance in the same events by American children as reported in numerous studies (Espenschade, 1960) illustrates both these types of variations.

The jumps used in the two sets of data are of different types and are, therefore, not numerically comparable. However, an examination of the growth curves shows a consistent increase in all types of jumps for the males of both countries until the later adolescent years when there is a slight leveling off. In the American data for jumps, a marked leveling off occurs after the 13th year for girls, while a similar leveling off does not occur in the Bulgarian girls until the 16th year. Data for the run and distance throw are comparable upon conversion of the metric system to yards and feet. Table 12 gives the average performance scores in the distance throw for boys and girls of both countries in the overlapping age ranges and Figure 65 illustrates similar averages for the run.

An examination of Table 12 indicates that the American boys and girls have preadolescent increments in performance which enable them to exceed their Bulgarian counterparts, whereas performances for the two groups were either comparable or slightly better for the Bulgarians before and after these increments. Ages in which performances of the American girls exceed the Bulgarian are 9 and 10 years, while performances of the American boys exceed the Bulgarian at 10, 11, and 12 years. It may be recalled that menarche occurs sooner in American girls than in European girls (Shuttle-

Table 12
Comparison of Bulgarian[a] and American[b] Performance
Scores in Distance Throw in Feet*

Age	Boys		Girls	
	Bulgarian	American	Bulgarian	American
8	65.0	57.4	32.5	30.0
9	72.8	66.6	36.8	38.7
10	81.3	83.0	42.3	47.0
11	90.5	95.0	55.8	54.0
12	101.0	104.0	61.7	61.0
13	114.5	114.0	68.2	70.0
14	123.4	123.0	75.1	74.5
15	131.6	135.0	82.0	75.7
16	145.7	144.0	86.3	74.0
17	162.4	153.0		

* [a]Based on data from Ivan Mangarov, "Physical Development and Capacity of Bulgarian Students". *Bulletin d'Information, Bulgarian Olympic Committee,* Year IX, No. 5:22-28, 1964.

* [b]From *Science and Medicine of Exercise and Sports,* edited by Warren R. Johnson: Copyright © 1960 by Warren R. Johnson: "Motor Development" by Anna Espenschade. Reprinted by permission of Harper & Row, Publishers.

worth, 1949) and earlier increments in performance may reflect this difference. Table 12 also indicates that the performance of American girls declines after the age of 15 whereas the Bulgarian girls' performance is still increasing.

Similarly, Figure 65 indicates faster running scores for American boys until 17 years of age when Bulgarian boys equal their performance, and for American girls until 15 years when Bulgarian girls equal and subsequently surpass their performance level. The Bulgarian performance curves for the run are complicated by different distances from ages 8 to 11 inclusive and from 12 to 18 years. At the younger ages the 40 meter dash was used while the 60 meter dash was standard for the remaining ages. This discrepancy in distance may account for the lower scores of the Bulgarian children, in comparison with the American, from 9 to 11 years, and for the sharp increase in yards per second between 11 and 12 years, since the relative weighting of the start will have less effect on the time in

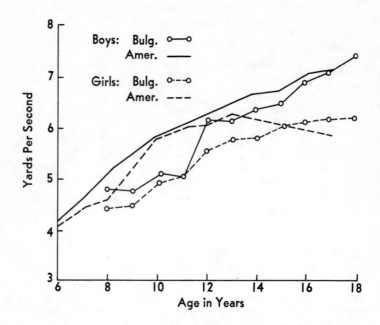

Figure 65.   Curves of running performance for Bulgarian
                  and American boys and girls. (Adapted from
                  Bulgarian data by Ivan Mangarov, "Physical
                  Development and Capacity of Bulgarian
                  Students." **Bulletin d'Information, Bulgarian
                  Olympic Committee,** Year IX, No. 5:22-28,
                  1964. Adapted from American data by Anna
                  Espenschade, "Motor Development." In
                  Warren R. Johnson (Ed.), **Science and Medi-
                  cine of Exercise and Sports.** New York:
                  Harper & Row, Publishers, 1960.)

the longer run. Even with approximately comparable distances in
the run, however, American girls equal the performance of Bulgarian boys at 12 and 13 years, following which time the American
girls decline steadily.

It would appear, then, that regional variation in performance
of basic motor skills is conditioned by some of the same factors that

influence growth until the age of puberty, after which time cultural influences play an increasingly prominent role in motor performance.

In summary, changes in body size and physique and in biological and physiological functioning are very marked in boys during adolescence. The increased leverage, strength, and endurance associated with these changes result in large improvements in performance in all motor activities. Although girls have equally as marked changes in body physique and biological functioning, the changes associated with body size and physiological functioning are not as great as in boys. Furthermore, increments in leverage, strength, and endurance are less than for boys while some of the changes in body physique may actually be detrimental to performance in some activities. Therefore, performances in girls tend to level off, and in some instances decline, with the advent of the menarche.

Cultural influences also play a role in the more marked differentiation of performance levels between the sexes at puberty. The American culture encourages participation in sporting and athletic events for males but does not do so for females, especially during adolescence and adulthood. Therefore, the performance scores for males are secured in a culturally approving environment, whereas the averages for females are based upon culturally indifferent, or discouraged, performance.

CHAPTER X

PERFORMANCE IN ADULTHOOD AND OLD AGE

Following the period of rapid adolescent development there is a period of gradual increase in size and capacity and finally a leveling off or plateau in adulthood when few growth changes occur. Increments in physical performance are now due to practice, training, experience, and interest. The basic performances of childhood, running, jumping, and throwing, are no longer commonly engaged in by large numbers of individuals so that there is little available data comparable to that of the growing years.

However, the AAHPER Youth Fitness Test Manual gives norms, based upon scores from thousands of individuals, for various events from the age of 10 years to college level. A comparison of the 50th percentile scores of 17-year-old boys and girls with college men and women indicates a general superiority of the college groupings over the 17-year-olds. Table 13 shows that college women are superior in performance in sit-ups, shuttle run, standing broad jump, 50-yard dash, and 600-yard run-walk, whereas performance in modified pull-up and softball throw is slightly lower. Similarly, Table 14

lists college men as being superior in all items except pull-ups and
50-yard dash, but even here the norms are identical.

Table 13
50th Percentile Scores for Women in Various Fitness Test Items*

Age	17 years	College
Modified Pull-ups	21	20
Sit-ups	16	20
Shuttle Run (Sec.)	11.8	11.6
Standing Broad Jump	5' 0"	5' 4"
50-Yard Dash (Sec.)	8.6	8.4
Softball Throw (Ft.)	79	70
600-Yard Run-Walk (Min.)	3:11	2:58

* Adapted from *AAHPER Youth Fitness Test Manual*. Washington, D.C.:
American Association for Health, Physical Education and Recreation, 1961. By
permission of the publisher.

Table 14
50th Percentile Scores for Men in Various Fitness Test Items**

Age	17 years	College
Pull-ups	6	6
Sit-ups	44	47
Shuttle Run (Sec.)	10.3	9.7
Standing Broad Jump	6' 11"	7' 3"
50-Yard Dash (Sec.)	6.8	6.8
Softball Throw (Ft.)	176	184
600-Yard Run-Walk (Min.)	2:04	1:52

** Adapted from *AAHPER Youth Fitness Test Manual*. Washington, D.C.:
American Association for Health, Physical Education and Recreation, 1961. By
permission of the publisher.

A study of physical fitness of Army Air Force personnel indicates
a decline in performance for various test items after the age of 21
years (Larson, 1946). Here a steady decline was noted in 60-yard
dash, sit-ups, chinning, standing broad jump, squat-thrust (Burpee)
test, and 360-yard run for men from 21 to 48 years with the physical

fitness rating, based upon all test items, showing a similar decline. Men in this study were highly motivated and without doubt represented a selected sample of the total population. Thus the decrease in scores should be thought of as representative of adult males in good physical condition.

CHANGES IN STRENGTH AND MUSCULATURE

The musculature of the body, as the only volitional means by which the body is capable of movement, is a vital factor mediating performance and the amount of work the body can accomplish. Figure 66 indicates a consistent loss in dominant hand grip strength in males after the age of 22 years so that the 80-year-old man is, on the average, not as strong as the 13-year-old boy. The decline is most marked after the age of 35 years, when there is a drop from 44 kilograms to 23 kilograms at 90 years of age in dominant hand grip (Shock, 1962).

Patterns of decline in strength of the dominant and subordinate hand are similar for the sexes, with the dominant hand being stronger at all ages than the subordinate hand but losing a greater amount of strength with increased age in comparison with the subordinate hand (Miles, 1950). A survey of a number of research studies by Welford (1959) indicates that other areas of the body show similar percentages of decline in strength of the musculature with increased age. However, the loss of grip endurance, namely the amount that can be held for one minute, is not nearly as great as that of grip strength with the 75-year-old man having, on the average, a higher grip-strength endurance than the 13-year-old boy (Figure 66). From a grip strength of 28 kilograms at 20 years the decline is only 8 kilograms over the intervening years to age 75 (Shock, 1962).

The loss of strength may be explained partly by the reduction of androgen production in males but such an explanation would not account for a similar reduction on the part of females. Perhaps an explanation may lie in the increase in collagen which fills up the spaces between muscle fibers as the individual grows older. Such "dead" material added to the muscle structure would tend to reduce the effective strength of the muscle. Furthermore, the molecular

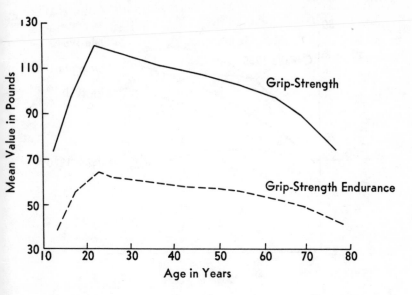

Figure 66.   Changes with age in dominant hand grip and grip-strength endurance in males. (From W. E. Burke, W. W. Tuttle, C. W. Thompson, C. D. Janney and R. J. Weber, "The Relation of Grip Strength and Grip-Strength Endurance to Age." **J. appl. Physiol.**, 5:628-630, 1953. By permission of the authors and publisher.)

changes that collagen undergoes as it ages produce stiff joints and leathery skin in the aged (Verzár, 1963). The less resilient skin of the aged (Shock, 1952) and the hampering effects of less moveable and flexible joints would tend to further reduce the effective strength of the musculature.

PHYSICAL SIZE AND MOTOR PERFORMANCE

The secular trend of increased height and weight during childhood and adolescence is reflected in increased stature and weight

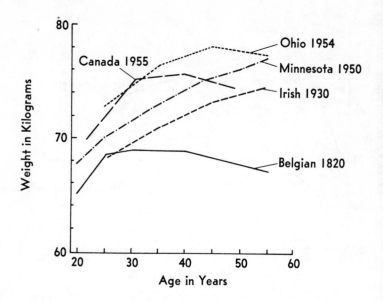

Figure 67.   Age-weight trends for five male populations,
                    1820 to 1955. (From S. M. Garn, "Fat Accu-
                    mulation and Aging in Males and Females."
                    In B. L. Strehler, Editor, **The Biology of Ag-
                    ing.** Washington, D. C.: American Institute
                    of Biological Sciences, 1960. By permission of
                    the editor and publisher.)

during adulthood. Data on Norwegian adults shows little gain
height from 1760 to 1830 but hereafter gains about 1.5 cm. (0.3
cm./decade) from 1830 to 1875 and approximately 4 cm. (0.6
cm./decade) between 1876 and 1935 (Kiil, 1939). Similarly, the average height of American enlisted men increased from 67.5 inches to
68.1 inches from World War I to World War II (Jones and Jones,
1957). The trend toward increased weight for adults of both sexes
is illustrated in Figures 67 and 68.

Such a secular trend toward increased body size in adulthood

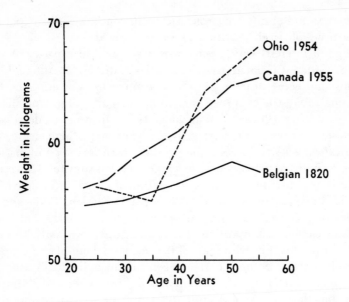

Figure 68. Age-weight trends for three female populations, 1820 to 1955. (From S. M. Garn, "Fat
Accumulation and Aging in Males and Females." In B. L. Strehler, Editor, **The Biology
of Aging.** Washington, D. C.: American Institute of Biological Sciences, 1960. By permission of the editor and publisher.)

should have some effect upon motor performance. Unfortunately,
no long range data are available for average adult performance and
the limited data on adolescents indicates that cultural influences
may play a large role in average performance (Espenschade and
Meleney, 1961; Hunsicker and Reiff, 1966). However, the constant
improvement in world records by champion athletes over the years
would certainly indicate that body size is important in this, in
addition to advances that have been made in training methods,
performance techniques, and equipment.

INTEREST AND PHYSICAL ACTIVITY

Interest and ability are strong factors in continuing participation in various physical activities. However, over the years there is a change in interests which reflects reduced physical capacity. A decline in interest is noted in such activities as driving an automobile, tennis, and being pitted against another in politics or athletics. Increasing interest is expressed in visiting museums, observing birds, and gardening (Pressey and Kuhlen, 1957). In general, decreased interest is expressed in those activities requiring a high degree of physical capacity and stress, whereas there is an increased liking for those activities which are more sedentary and less stressful. However, there is also a decreased liking for continual changing of activities as the individual grows older (Pressey and Kuhlen, 1957) and a survey of 2,340 men, ranging in age from 20 to 59 years, indicates that the change in proportion of likes and dislikes was only 7.5 percent during this time with most of the changes taking place between 25 and 35 years (Strong, 1931). In general, an individual's activity participation tends to remain fairly stable (Desroches and Kaiman, 1964) but there are very definite differences in activity patternings within various socio-economic groupings (Heyman and Jeffers, 1964).

Interest in an activity would appear to be strongly conditioned by one's facility in the particular activity. Reduction of interest in driving an automobile may, in part, be attributed to decreased skill, on the basis of bad records and blame for accidents on the part of drivers over 60 years of age (McFarland et al., 1964). Furthermore, aging athletes have a significantly lower participation record in athletic activities than do older non-athletes (Montoye et al., 1957). In this instance, although the athlete may still have a slightly higher level of performance at all ages than the non-athlete, his decline in proficiency is obviously greater in comparison to his peak performance and consequently satisfaction may not be obtained from what, to him, is an inferior performance.

Studies such as that of Younger (1959), which deals with reaction and movement times, have explored the differences between athletes and non-athletes and found athletes to be slightly superior. It was previously mentioned, in the chapter dealing with heredity, that reaction and movement times are genetically mediated to a high degree and it is also likely that balance, kinesthetic perception, and motor coordination are similarly determined to a great extent by heredity. Practice, training, and experience can increase performance only to the limits of innate motor ability. Thus, the highly skilled athlete achieves his stature because he has a high degree of native endowment in these areas and develops his skills to their optimal potential.

PEAK PHYSICAL PERFORMANCE

If one regards championship performance as indicative of peak proficiency in an activity, then, according to Table 15, the range of such performance is 22 to 35 years. However, the recent performances of young swimmers, particularly women, would indicate that the lower limits of peak proficiency should be extended to around 15 years. In general, peak proficiency is attained at an earlier age in those activities requiring strength, speed, and endurance, whereas championship performance is more common at the later ages in relatively less vigorous activities where experience is also a factor.

It is possible to compare the results in Table 15 with the ages at which 1,359 superior contributions were made by 933 individuals in the fields of science, mathematics, and practical invention. In each instance, to reduce the curves to a comparable basis, proper allowance is made for the mortality rate, and the age at which the greatest number of contributions are made is set at 100 percent. The contributions at other ages are proportionally adjusted to this standard. Figure 69 indicates that the age of maximum proficiency in all 17 physical skills listed in Table 15 occurs approximately 4 years before the age of maximal number of superior contributions in the scientific fields. Furthermore, the curve of championship contributions in physical achievement falls away much more abruptly from the optimal age at 30 years than does that for the contributions in the scientific fields.

However, when a comparison is made with age of maximal proficiency in five physical activities involving fine neuromuscular coordination and precision of movement rather than vigorous per-

Table 15
Ages at which individuals have exhibited proficiency at "physical" skills*

Type of skill	No. of cases	Median age	Mean age	Years of maximum proficiency
U.S.A. outdoor tennis champions	89	26.35	27.12	22-26
Runs batted in: annual champions of the two major baseball leagues	49	27.10	27.97	25-29
U.S.A. indoor tennis champions	64	28.00	27.45	25-29
World champion heavy-weight pugilists	77	29.19	29.51	26-30
Base stealers: annual champions of the two major baseball leagues	31	29.21	28.85	26-30
Indianapolis-Speedway racers and national auto-racing champions	82	29.56	30.18	27-30
Best hitters: annual champions of the two major baseball leagues	53	29.70	29.56	27-31
Best pitchers: annual champions of the two major baseball leagues	51	30.10	30.03	28-32
Open golf champions of England and of the U.S.A.	127	30.72	31.29	28-32
National individual rifle-shooting champions	84	31.33	31.45	32-34
State corn-husking champions of the U.S.A.	103	31.50	30.66	28-31
World, national, and state pistol-shooting champions	47	31.90	30.63	31-34
National amateur bowling champions	58	32.33	32.78	30-34
National amateur duck-pin bowling champions	91	32.35	32.19	30-34
Professional golf champions of England and of the U.S.A.	53	32.44	32.14	29-33
World record-breakers at billiards	42	35.00	35.67	30-34
World champion billiardists	74	35.75	34.38	31-35

* From Harvey C. Lehman, *Age and Achievement.* Published for the American Philosophical Society by Princeton University Press, Princeton, 1953, p. 256. By permission of the American Philosophical Society.

234

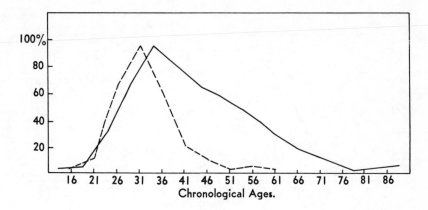

Figure 69. Age versus output in science and proficiency in certain vigorous skills. Solid line, scientific output. Broken line, 1,175 championships in 17 classes listed in Table 15. (From Harvey C. Lehman, **Age and Achievement.** Published for the American Philosophical Society by Princeton University Press, Princeton, 1953. By permission of the American Philosophical Society.)

formance, the age of maximal proficiency coincides with that of the maximal number of superior contributions in the scientific fields, although the rate of decline in maintenance of such performance remains much steeper (Figure 70). A further comparison of proficiency in billiards, a fine neuromuscular skill, with output in chemistry indicates an identical age of maximal proficiency and very similar curves for performance at other age levels (Figure 71). The surprising similarity of curves of proficiency in billiards and outstanding contributions in chemistry is not the only instance of such a relationship between activities which are primarily of a physical nature and those that are considered to be in the realm of the intellectual. Similar curves are also found for football professionalism and lyric writing and for proficiency in billiards and golf and oil painting (Lehman. 1953).

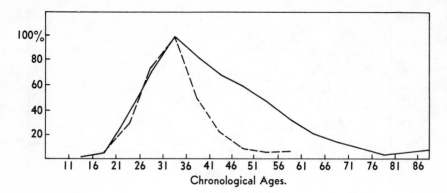

Chronological Ages.

Figure 70.   Age versus output in science and proficiency in certain skills. Solid line, scientific output. Broken line, 577 championships at golf, billiards, rifle and pistol shooting, bowling, and duck-pin bowling—skills of the nicest neuromuscular coordination. (From Harvey C. Lehman, **Age and Achievement.** Published for the American Philosophical Society by Princeton University Press, Princeton, 1953. By permission of the American Philosophical Society.)

One may also consider geographical discoveries and explorations to require both a high degree of intellectual capacity and physical proficiency. Graphing such achievements with output in science reveals remarkably similar curves. Figure 72 indicates that peak performances in geographical exploration and output in science coincide, and the slope of the declining performance in both areas is very similar.

It would appear, therefore, that optimal performance in very vigorous physical activities is the domain of the young adult. However, high levels of performance may be maintained over a longer period of time in those activities requiring a lesser degree of vigorous functioning but with a high degree of fine neuromuscular coordina-

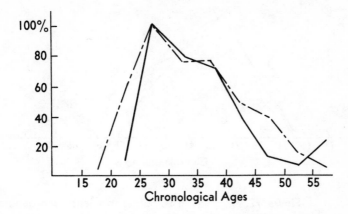

Figure 71. Age versus output in chemistry and proficiency in billiards. Solid line, 52 greatest chemical contributions of all time (selected by three university chemistry teachers). Broken line, 136 professional championships at billiards. (From Harvey C. Lehman, **Age and Achievement.** Published for the American Philosophical Society by Princeton University Press, Princeton, 1953. By permission of the American Philosophical Society.)

tion and precision of movement. Moreover, there is a marked similarity in performance curves for areas which require a superior physical capacity, but not necessarily championship performance, and contributions in various scientific, literary, and artistic fields.

ATHLETES AND LONGEVITY

It would appear, then, that interest and liking, conditioned by socio-economic factors, play equally important roles in actual individual physical capacity in motor performance during adulthood and old age. Such a complexity of factors make any assessment of

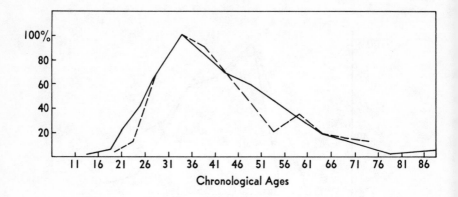

Figure 72.   Age versus output in science and geographical exploration. Solid line, scientific output. Broken line, 202 geographical explorations and discoveries (including polar expeditions) by 152 persons, now deceased, averaging 1.33 achievements per individual. (From Harvey C. Lehman, **Age and Achievement.** Published for the American Philosophical Society by Princeton University Press, Princeton, 1953. By permission of the American Philosophical Society.)

the influence of exercise upon retardation of aging and upon longevity exceedingly difficult and decidedly conjectural. A comparison of college athletes with non-athletes attending the same institution at the same time indicated little difference in the longevity of the two groups nor was there any difference in the longevity of the parents of the two groups (Montoye et al., 1957). Results of a similar study of records of 38,269 college men, of whom 6,492 were honor men and 4,976 athletes, were tabulated in terms of life expectancy and mortality rates in Table 16. Similar statistics are also recorded for the white male population in the United States over the same period of time.

Table 16
Expectancy of life and mortality rates per 1,000 of college graduates compared with white males in the United States in 1900-1902*

Age	College Graduates	Athletes	Honor men	United States white males 1900-1902
Life Expectancy				
22	45.71	45.56	47.73	40.71
42	29.44	28.92	31.07	26.33
62	14.48	14.09	15.56	13.17
82	4.56	4.24	4.98	4.54
Mortality Rate per 1,000				
22	4.38	4.04	3.68	6.68
42	6.26	6.12	5.11	11.24
62	26.14	26.39	22.10	32.76
82	138.30	151.16	123.08	155.42

* From Louis I. Dublin, Alfred J. Lotka, and Mortimer Spiegelman. *Length of Life*. New York: The Ronald Press Company, 1949. By permission of the publisher.

Athletes differ little from the general college population with respect to life expectancy and mortality rates, while honor college graduates have a slight advantage in these areas over the average college student and athlete. College graduates as a whole have a decided advantage in life expectancy and mortality rate in comparison with the entire white male population of the same age grouping. College graduates in general, and honor men in particular, achieve a higher socio-economic status than the population as a whole and a very definite relationship has been found between socio-economic status and death rate.

FACTORS AFFECTING LIFE SPAN

The longevity of an individual is influenced by the same factors that bear a relationship to growth, namely: heredity, sex, socio-economic status, race, geographic area, and temporal era. The records of 3,000,000 men insured with 34 American and Canadian companies were categorized into those individuals whose parents both lived to age 75 and those whose parents both died under the age of 60 years (Dublin et al., 1949). Figure 73 indicates that the mortality of the men with long-lived parents was distinctly lower than that of the group whose parents had died before the age of 60 years, with the difference averaging 20 percent. At 27 years of age, the individuals with long-lived parents had a life expectancy of 2⅓ years more than those with short-lived parents. Lansing (1959), in a comprehensive discussion of the biology of senescence, contends there is an extensive collection of data supporting an heritable component to longevity.

The previously mentioned greater propensity of females for survival at all ages is reflected in longer life spans in comparison with males. In 1952, a white man of 64 years could look forward to 13 years of life, whereas a white woman of the same age had a life expectancy of 15¾ years (Wilson, 1957). Negro females also have a higher survival rate and, consequently, longer life span than Negro males but it is not until the age of 82 years that the survival rate of Negro females equals and subsequently surpasses white males to result in a longer life span (Comfort, 1964).

The lower survival rates of Negro females up to the age of 82 in comparison with white males, yet with longer life spans, suggest that socio-economic factors may, in part, be influencing these data. Table 17 indicates there is a rise in mortality rate with decreasing socio-economic levels. The occupational groupings which have a high percentage of college graduates, namely, professional, technical, administrative, and managerial workers, have the lower ratio of death rates from ages 20 to 64 years. It may also be argued that the occupations having the higher mortality rate, such as semiskilled workers and laborers, also have specific hazards which outweigh socio-economic levels. However, the same pattern was observed in a British study in which wives were classified on the basis of occupation of their husbands and, from this, it may be inferred that mortality is influenced more by socio-economic environment than by occupational hazards (Spiegelman, 1960).

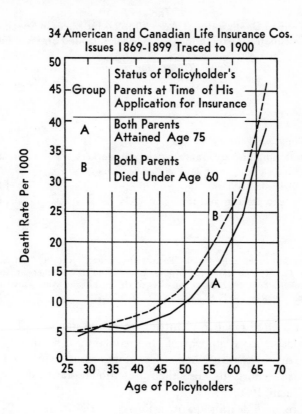

34 American and Canadian Life Insurance Cos.
Issues 1869-1899 Traced to 1900

Figure 73.   Death rates at successive ages among white
male policyholders classified according to
longevity of parents. (From Louis I. Dublin,
Alfred J. Lotka and Mortimer Spiegelman,
Length of Life. New York: The Ronald Press
Company, 1949. By permission of the publisher.)

Similarly, a survey of the death rates in a large number of countries shows the death rate to be much lower, or conversely the survival rate to be much higher, in countries with better socio-economic
conditions. It also indicates that the decline in death rate since 1920

Table 17
Ratio of Death Rates at Ages 20 to 64 for Males in Specified Occupation Level to that for All Males, United States, 1950*

Occupation Level	Ratio of death rate to all males
All males	1.00
Professional workers	.84
Technical, administrative and managerial workers	.87
Proprietors, clerical, sales, and skilled workers	.96
Semiskilled workers	1.00
Laborers, except farm and mine	1.65
Agricultural workers	.88

* From Mortimer Spiegelman, "Factors in Human Mortality." In Bernard L. Strehler, Editor, *The Biology of Aging.* Washington, D.C.: American Institute of Biological Sciences, 1960. By permission of the editor and American Institute of Biological Sciences.

has not been as great in countries where the standard of living has been consistently high, whereas the reduction in death rate is quite marked in areas which had a low standard of living in 1920 but have made efforts to raise their nutritional standards since then (Spiegelman, 1960).

The reduced death rates in various countries from 1920-24 to 1959 indicate a secular trend toward greater life expectancy. Such is indeed the case and there has been a decided increase in life expectancy over the centuries since ancient Grecian times (Figure 74). The rapid improvement in life span following the middle of the 19th century coincides with the rapid increases in medical knowledge and improvements in socio-economic conditions brought about by the industrial revolution. Therefore, increased life span over the centuries is based upon reduced death rates rather than any noted change in inheritable longevity. Wilson (1957) indicates that, over the past four decades, the death rate for all ages decreased for both white males and white females in the United States. This decline in death rate is also consistently greater for females than for males in that life expectancy for males was increased $18\frac{1}{3}$ years from 1900 to

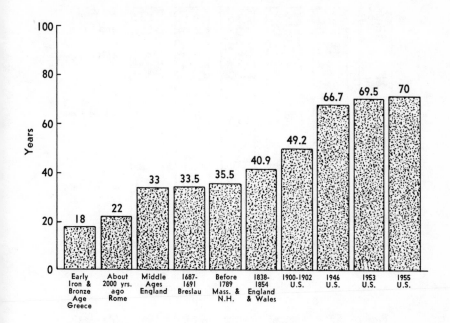

Figure 74.   Average length of life from ancient Greece to modern times. (From Otto von Mering and Frederick L. Weniger, "Social-Cultural Background of the Aging Individual." In J. E. Birren, Editor, **Handbook of Aging and the Individual.** Chicago: The University of Chicago Press, 1959. By permission of the publisher.)

1951, whereas it was raised by 21½ years for females over the same time span.

The increases in life span of the population have resulted in shifts in the proportion of individuals within selected age groupings. The population structure of the United States at various times from 1860 to the estimated percentage grouping in 1980 is depicted in Figure 75. The most dominant trend is the increasing proportion of the population within the 45 year and older age groupings. These

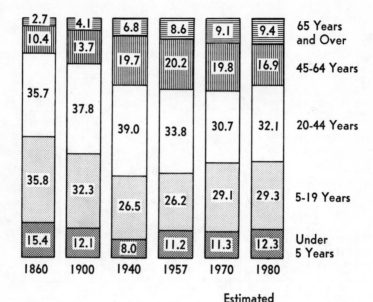

2.7	4.1	6.8	8.6	9.1	9.4	65 Years and Over
10.4	13.7	19.7	20.2	19.8	16.9	45-64 Years
35.7	37.8	39.0	33.8	30.7	32.1	20-44 Years
35.8	32.3	26.5	26.2	29.1	29.3	5-19 Years
15.4	12.1	8.0	11.2	11.3	12.3	Under 5 Years
1860	1900	1940	1957	1970	1980	

Estimated

Figure 75.   Population structure of the United States by percentage of the population in selected age groups. (From Otto von Mering and Frederick L. Weniger, "Social-Cultural Background of the Aging Individual." In J. E. Birren, Editor, **Handbook of Aging and the Individual.** Chicago: The University of Chicago Press, 1959. By permission of the publisher.)

percentage gains are mainly at the expense of the 5 to 44 year age groupings where the percentage decline may be a result of war-time casualties and the trend toward smaller families prior to 1940.

CHANGES ASSOCIATED WITH AGING

With an increasing proportion of the population in the age groupings of 45 years or older and the general increase in life expectancy, the study of aging, or gerontology, has become one of the major areas of research dealing with human development. Because of the recency of concentration on the problems of aging and the difficulties associated with longitudinal studies of human beings, the majority of research studies in this area are based upon cross-sectional data.

The primary mechanism in aging is considered by Bjorksten (1963) to be the phenomenon of cross-linking between the giant molecules of the body, in particular the proteins and nucleic acids, with somatic mutations, loss of elasticity, and accumulation of immobilized material being of secondary importance. Cross-linkage is favored as the primary mechanism because it is the only known process by which a single small molecule can drastically change the behavior of two giant molecules; and because the known number of cross-linking agents normally present in the body is so great the occurrence of cross-linkages, including the irreversible type, is inescapable.

On the other hand, other investigators express the opinion that no single mechanism seems to cause aging, although there appears to be a progression in which genetically controlled metabolism may be involved (Sullivan et al., 1963). According to Shock (1962), youth is marked by tremendous reserves in all the organs of the body, whereas the aging process involves the progressive loss of body tissue from the muscles, nervous system, and many vital organs which result in increasing loss of reserve. There are great variations in the rate of loss of different functions among individuals and within each individual with respect to various aspects of function.

Structural changes and a general decline in physiological functioning accompany increases in age after 30 years. The changes associated with strength and muscular structure have already been mentioned. Similarly, there are changes in the work rate of an individual with increased age. Figure 76 indicates that maximum work rate over a sustained period of time, based on a two-step climbing test, reaches its optimal level in females around the age of 25 years, while peak work performance in males occurs around 28 years of age. Following the achievement of optimal performance, there is a continuous gradual decline in work rate which is slightly greater in males than in females, so that the work differential between the sexes becomes less with increasing age.

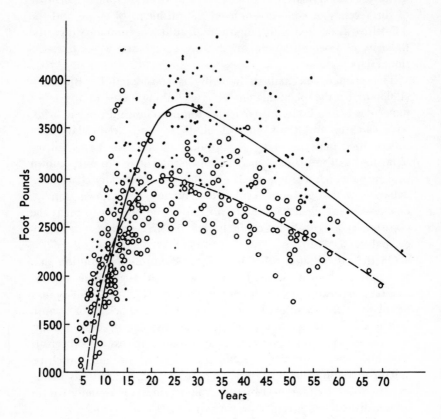

Figure 76. Relation of age to exercise tolerance as expressed in foot pounds of work per minute. Straight line (through dots) for male and broken line (through circles) for female individuals. (From A. M. Master, "The Two-Step Test of Myocardial Function." **Amer. Heart J.,** 10:495-510, 1935. By permission of the publisher, The C. V. Mosby Company, St. Louis.)

Although the maximum sustained work rate drops approximately 30 percent from 500 kilogram-meters per minute at 30 years to 350 kilogram-meters per minute in a 70-year-old man, there is an even greater decline during short periods of rapid work. The maximum work rate for short bursts of work on the hand ergometer falls from 1,850 kilogram-meters per minute in 35-year-old men to 750 kilogram meters for 80-year-olds—a decline of almost 60 percent (Shock, 1962). Increasing age, therefore, results in a reduced tolerance range toward physical activity as well as reduced capacity for such activity. This reduction in both range and capacity may readily be explained in terms of reduced physiological functioning in general.

Cardiac output is, of course, a significant factor in the speed of transmission of food and oxygen to areas of muscular activity and in the removal of products of such activity. Cross-sectional studies indicate a consistent decline in the highest heart rate that can be attained during maximal work with increasing age (Robinson, 1938). Longitudinal studies also show such decline in varying amounts (Dawson and Hellebrandt, 1945; Dill, 1942, 1958). The heart rate is linearly correlated with the intensity of exercise in terms of net oxygen consumption for both young and old men (Aghemo et al., 1964), but old subjects have a greater heart response during submaximal work (Norris et al., 1953) and show a delayed circulatory recuperation following exercise (Norris and Shock, 1960).

Blood circulation time is significantly prolonged in men over 70 years in comparison with the norm for young men (Diettert, 1963). However, a comparison of red blood cells and blood volumes of men over 70 years with norms of young males indicates little difference (Hurdle and Rosin, 1962). Moreover, body size, heart volume, and blood volume are not significantly correlated with maximum heart rate or maximal work in old men (Strandell, 1964), indicating that physical working capacity in old men may be limited by either vascular or muscular-metabolic peripheral factors.

Collagenous changes in the structure of various organs is undoubtedly also a factor in their reduced functioning with increasing age. The heart muscle of the rat has been found to have an almost three fold increase in the collagen concentration with age (Schaub, 1964/5). These results, coupled with the findings of Kohn and Rollerson (1959) of reduction in the swelling ability of the human heart with age, suggest that the addition of collagen to the muscle tissue reduces the structural flexibility and imposes an additional load on the contracting heart muscle.

The respiratory system shows a reduction in vital capacity, maximum ventilation volume during exercise, maximum voluntary breathing capacity, and maximum oxygen uptake during exercise with increasing age. The decline in vital capacity from 30 to 80 years is 40 percent, while the reduction in maximum breathing capacity is almost 60 percent (Figure 77). Ventilation responses of young males are also larger during early adjustment to exercise than they are for older subjects (Norris and Shock, 1960).

The reduced blood flow undoubtedly accounts for part of the reduced oxygen uptake (Shock, 1962). However, the reduction in blood flow alone does not seem to account for the great difference in oxygen uptake between the young and the old. The arterial oxygen and percentage saturation in elderly individuals are also low, indicating either unequal ventilation of the lungs or reduced diffusing capacity or both (Dill et al., 1963). On the basis of the great changes that occur in total lung capacity and in expiration reserve volume with aging, Norman et al. (1964) concluded that a state of mild chronic obstructive emphysema occurs in old age, whereas Edge et al. (1964) contend that aged lungs show only a mild degree of emphysema. Study of the chest X-rays of 100 subjects of 75 years or over led the latter investigators to the conclusion that there is no senile lung pattern, although decalcification of the ribs is generally present and there is some shrinkage of the thoracic cage. It is highly likely that no one factor is entirely accountable for reduction in pulmonary function and that various factors may account for varying degrees of function loss in different individuals.

Exercise tolerance is also affected by the ability of the body to remove waste products other than the carbon dioxide removed by the lungs. This is the function of the kidneys and Figure 77 indicates that the renal plasma flow and glomerular filtration rate are reduced approximately 50 percent. The maximum excretory capacity and glucose reabsorption capacity are also reduced to a similar extent. The slowing down of waste product removal is quite considerable between 30 and 80 years since there is a loss of 83 percent in the speed of return to equilibrium of blood acidity following exercise (Shock, 1962).

The integrity of the nervous system is vital to the initiation and coordination of muscular responses. There is a decrease, particularly

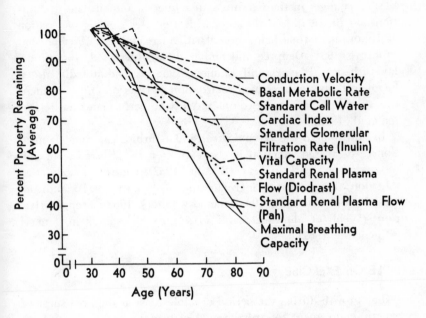

Figure 77.   Decline of various human functional capacities and physiological measurements with age. (From Bernard L. Strehler, Editor, **The Biology of Aging.** Washington, D. C.: American Institute of Biological Sciences, 1960. By permission of the editor and publisher.)

in the lumbosacral regions, in the number of fibers with each decade of life (Corbin and Gardner, 1937) which amounts to a reduction of 27 percent in the number of nerve trunk fibers with advanced age (Shock, 1962). Brain autopsy reveals a reduction in brain weight from 1,375 grams (3.03 lbs.) at 30 years to 1,232 grams (2.72 lbs.) at 90 years (Shock, 1962), while histological examination of the spinal cord shows degeneration which includes demyelinization and loss of nerve cells (Graux et al., 1962). Nerve conduction velocity loss is more prominent in distal segments of the body than in proximal areas (Mayer, 1963) and is greater in inferior parts of the body than in the superior members or the trunk (Graux et al., 1962).

Such changes in the nervous system suggest impairment of function and this is indeed the case, with a greater slowing of reaction and movement time being noted with increased age (Pierson and Montoye, 1958; Deupree and Simon, 1963). Increased synaptic delay with age (Wayner and Emmers, 1958) is undoubtedly also a factor in the noted increased retardation of reaction and movement times with the increasing complexity of the performance task (Birren et al., 1962).

In addition to the physiological and neurological changes mentioned, decreased function is also exhibited in adjustment to and recovery from work in heat (Brouha, 1962); control of body sway (Sheldon, 1963); pain (Sherman and Robillard, 1964); auditory sensitivity (Schaie et al., 1964); memory (Shock, 1962); sleep deprivation (Webb et al., 1962); and to sensory thresholds in general (Hinchcliffe, 1962).

ROLE OF EXERCISE

The growth during the period of adolescence is the final surge of genetic endowment toward the goal of a biologically mature individual, and any increments in performance subsequent to the cessation of growth are confined to the limits established at the termination of growth. With some individuals the range of limits is much greater than with others but this, too, is a feature of the numerous differences that make each individual unique. A good example of an extreme range of limits within one individual is that of Wilma Rudolph, who overcame a crippling condition in her legs during childhood to attain her optimal physical performance by becoming the fastest woman runner in the world during the 1960 Olympics.

Young adulthood, between 20 and 30 years, marks the period of optimal physical achievement for the average individual, although championship performance is not uncommon at a later age in those activities involving a high degree of experience. The individual then faces the slow, but inevitable, decline in physical and physiological functioning termed aging which, barring previous decease due to illness or accident, eventually results in the death of the individual. The rate at which this decline occurs appears to be greatly influenced by the amount of physical activity of the individual. Longitudinal data on Dill (1942, 1958) shows that he maintained a high level of physiological functioning with regular physical activity. Moreover, cross-sectional studies by Jokl (1954) indicate above-normal performance levels are maintained over the years by individuals who partake regularly in vigorous physical activity.

Numerous studies indicate the beneficial effect of physical training upon motor ability (Landiss, 1955); physical fitness (Larson, 1946; Landiss, 1955); circulatory changes (Michael and Gallon, 1959; Golding, 1961; Rochelle, 1961); and strength changes (Clarke, Shay, and Mathews, 1955; Berger, 1962, 1963). Studies such as those by Larson (1946) and Sloan (1963) show a higher level of physical fitness for individuals who are professionally engaged in physical education. Army Air Force physical training instructors were found to have consistently higher physical fitness ratings from ages 21 to 35 in comparison with other Air Force personnel (Larson, 1946). Similarly, physical education majors, both men and women, had significantly higher physical fitness indexes than sophomore college men and women (Sloan, 1963).

Within occupations of similar socio-economic levels the amount of activity appears to be an operative factor contributing to health and mortality rate. A study was made of the incidence and severity of coronary heart disease in postal and transportation workers in England. The postal group was subdivided into letter carriers and office workers, while the transportation grouping was subdivided into the more physically active conductors and the more sedentary drivers. In both general groupings, the more physically active subgroupings had relatively less coronary heart disease, with such heart disease as did occur being of less severe condition (Morris et al., 1953). A similar study of railroad clerks and railroad switchmen conducted by the Laboratory of Physiological Hygiene at the University of Minnesota, with electrocardiographic tests taken before and after treadmill work, indicated a significantly lower incidence of abnormalities in the switchmen than in the clerks (Simonson, 1957).

The maintenance of a high level of physical fitness is endorsed by the American Medical Association and American Heart Association, and physical activities which will challenge each person within the limits of his capabilities are strongly recommended. With our high standard of living, obesity has become a major health problem. The mortality rate for men who are 30 percent overweight is more than 40 percent greater than for those of proper weight. The U.S. Public Health Service recommends physical exercise and diet to prevent and reduce accumulation of excess weight. Clearly, then, the maintenance of physical fitness is of definite value to the health and well-being of an individual. Certainly, also, the individual who takes part regularly in physical activities would have a better knowledge of his capabilities in this area thus alleviating, to some degree, the loss of confidence as well as the physical weakness that have been noted as concomitants of the aging process (Sheldon, 1950).

In general, adulthood marks the period of greatest variability in human physical performance, with levels of achievement being influenced by interest, socio-economic environment, and cultural patterns as well as by inherent ability. With increasing age there is a decrease in all human functions in varying degrees. Factors such as heredity, socio-economic level, and occupation are of prime importance in the rate of such decline and also in mortality rate. There is, however, some indication that physically active individuals maintain a higher level of performance in most functions with increasing age. The habits and attitudes as well as the skills developed during the growing years play a vital role in health, both mental and physical, of any individual throughout his entire life. Motor skills learned in childhood or youth provide the tools which encourage participation and provide enjoyment in vigorous activity in the adult years.

BIBLIOGRAPHY

AAHPER Youth Fitness Test Manual (1961) Washington, D.C.: American Association for Health, Physical Education and Recreation.

Acheson, R. M. (1954) A method of assessing skeletal maturity from radio-graphs. A report from the Oxford Child Health Survey. *J. Anat.,* 88:498-508.

—————, and C. W. Dupertuis (1957) The relationship between physique and rate of skeletal maturation in boys. *Hum. Biol.* 29:167-193.

Aghemo, P., D. Gsell, and F. Mangili (1964) The relation of work performance to heart rate in aged man. *Gerontologia,* 9(2):91-97.

Ames, L. B. (1937) The sequential patterning of prone progression in the human infant. *Genet. Psychol. Monogr.,* 19:409-460.

—————— (1949) Development of interpersonal smiling responses in the preschool years. *J. Genet. Psychol.,* 74:273-291.

Ashley Montagu, M. F. (1946) *Adolescent Sterility. A Study in the Comparative Physiology of the Infecundity of the Adult Organism in Mammals and Man.* Springfield: Charles C. Thomas.

—————— (1962) *Prenatal Influences.* Springfield: Charles C. Thomas.

Atkinson, R. K. (1925) A study of athletic ability of high school girls, *Amer. Phys. Educ. Rev.,* 30:389-399.

Bachman, J. C. (1961) Motor learning and performance as related to age and sex in two measures of balance coordination. *Res. Quart.* 32:123-137.

Bailey, S. W. (1937) An experimental study of the origin of lateral-line structures in embryonic and adult teleosts. *J. Exp. Zool.,* 76:187-234.

Baird, D. (1945) The influence of social and economic factors on still-births and neonatal deaths. *J. Obstet. Gynaec. (Brit.),* 527:217-234.

Bakwin, H., and R. M. Bakwin (1931) Body build in infants: II. The proportions of the external dimensions of the healthy infant during the first year of life. *J. Clin. Invest.,* 10:377-394.

_____, and _____ (1936) Growth of thirty-two external dimensions during the first year of life. *J. Pediat.*, 8:177-183.

_____, and T. W. Patrick (1944) The weight of Negro infants. *J. Pediat.*, 24:405-407.

Baldwin, B. T. (1926) Anthropometric measurements. In L. M. Terman (ed.), *Genetic Studies of Genius. Vol. I. Mental and Physical Traits of a Thousand Gifted Children.* Palo Alto: Stanford University Press.

Ballantyne, J. W. and F. J. Browne (1922) The problems of foetal postmaturity and prolongation of pregnancy. *J. Obstet. Gynaec. Brit. Emp.*, 29:177-238.

Barcroft, J., D. H. Barron, A. T. Cowie, and P. H. Forsham (1940) The oxygen supply of the foetal brain of the sheep and the effect of asphyxia on foetal respiratory movement. *J. Physiol.*, 97:338-346.

_____, and M. J. Karvonen (1948) Action of carbon dioxide and cyanide on fetal respiratory movements: Development of chemo-reflex in sheep. *J. Physiol. (London)*, 107:153-161.

Barker, R. G., and C. P. Stone (1936) Physical development in relation to menarcheal age in university women. *Hum. Biol.*, 8:198-222.

Barnes, L. L., G. Sperling, and C. M. McCay (1947) Bone growth in normal and retarded growth rats. *J. Gerontol.*, 2:240-243.

Barry, A. J., and T. K. Cureton (1961) Factorial analysis of physique and performance in prepubescent boys. *Res. Quart.* 32:283-300.

Barsanti, R. A. (1954) The relationship between leg strength and performance of elementary school girls in the dash and standing broad jump. Unpublished master's thesis, University of Wisconsin, Madison.

Bass, R. (1939) An analysis of the components of tests of semi-circular canal function and of static and dynamic balance. *Res. Quart.*, 10:33-52.

Bayer, M., and N. Bayley (1959) *Growth Diagnosis.* Chicago: Univ. of Chicago Press.

Bayley, N. A scale of motor development. Unpublished paper, Institute of Child Welfare, University of California, Berkeley.

_____ (1935) The development of motor abilities during the first three years. *Monogr. Soc. Res. Child Develpm.*, 1(1):1-26.

_____ (1936) *The California Infant Scale of Motor Development.* Berkeley: University of California Press.

_____ (1943) Size and body build of adolescents in relation to rate of skeletal maturing. *Child Develpm.*, 14:47-90.

_____, and L. M. Bayer (1946) The assessment of somatic androgyny. *Amer. J. Phys. Anthrop.*, 4 N.S.:433-461.

_____, and F. C. Davis (1935) Growth changes in bodily size and proportions during the first three years: A developmental study of sixty-one children by repeated measurements. *Biometrika*, 27:26-87.

Beasley, W. C. (1933) Visual pursuit in 109 white and 142 Negro newborn infants. *Child Develpm.*, 4:106-120.

Berger, R. (1962) Effect of varied weight training programs on strength. *Res. Quart.* 33(2):168-181.

———— (1963) Comparison between static training and various dynamic training programs. *Res. Quart.* 34(2):131-135.

Berry, W. T. C., P. J. Cowin, and H. E. Magee (1952) Haemoglobin levels in adults and children. *Brit. med. J.*, 1:410-412.

Birren, J. E., K. F. Riegel, and D. F. Morrison (1962) Age differences in response speed as a function of controlled variations of stimulus conditions: Evidence of a general speed factor. *Gerontologia*, 6(1):1-18.

Bjorksten, J. (1963) Aging, primary mechanism. *Gerontologia*, 8(2/3):179-192.

Blanton, M. G. (1917) The behavior of the human infant during the first thirty days of life. *Psychol. Rev.*, 24:456-483.

Boas, E. P., and E. F. Goldschmidt (1932) *The Heart Rate.* Springfield: Charles C. Thomas.

Bolaffio, M., and F. Artom (1924) Ricerche sulla fisiologia del sistema nervosa del feto umano. *Arch. sci. biol.*, 5:457-487.

Bolk, L. (1926) Untersuchungen uber die Menarche bei der niederlandischen Bevolkerung. *Z. Geburtsh. Gynak.*, 89:364-380.

Boynton, B. (1936) The physical growth of girls: A study of the rhythm of physical growth from anthropometric measurements on girls between birth and eighteen years. *Univ. Iowa Stud. Child Welfare*, 12(4):1-105.

Breckenridge, M. E., and E. L. Vincent (1949) *Child Development.* Philadelphia: Saunders.

Breitinger, Emil (1935) Body form and athletic achievement of youths. (Trans. and cond. by Ernst Thomas). *Res. quart.*, 6:83-91.

Bridgman, C. S., and L. Carmichael (1935) An experimental study of the onset of behavior in the fetal guinea-pig. *J. Genet. Psychol.*, 47:247-267.

Broman, B., G. Dahlberg, and A. Lichtenstein (1942) Height and weight during growth. *Acta. paediat. (Upsala)*, 30:1-66.

Brouha, L. (1962) Heat and the older worker. *J. Amer. Geriat. Soc.*, 10(1):35-39.

Burke, B. S., V. V. Harding, and H. C. Stuart (1943) Nutrition studies during pregnancy, relation of protein content of mother's diet during pregnancy to birth weight, length and condition of infant at birth. *J. Pediat.*, 23:506-515.

Burke, W. E., W. W. Tuttle, C. W. Thompson, C. D. Janney, and R. J. Weber (1953) The relation of grip strength and grip-strength endurance to age. *J. appl. Physiol.* 5:628-630.

Carlson, A. J., and H. Ginsburg (1915) Contributions to the physiology of the stomach. XXIV. The tonus and hunger contraction of the stomach of the newborn. *Amer. J. Physiol.*, 38:29-32.

Carmichael, L. (1951) Ontogenetic development. In Stevens, S. S. (ed.), *Handbook of Experimental Psychology.* New York: John Wiley & Sons, Inc.

_____ (1954) The onset and early development of behavior. In L. Carmichael, (ed.), *Manual of Child Psychology.* New York: John Wiley & Sons, Inc., Second Edition.

Carpenter, A. (1942a) The measurement of general motor capacity and general motor ability in the first three grades. *Res. Quart.* 13(4):444-465.

_____ (1942b) Strength in testing in the first three grades. *Res. Quart.,* 13:328-332.

Cearley, J. E. (1957) Linearity of contributions of ages, heights, and weights to prediction of track and field performances. *Res. Quart.,* 28:218-222.

Clarke, H. H. and G. H. Carter (1959) Oregon simplification of the strength and physical fitness indices. *Res. Quart.,* 30:3-10.

_____ and E. W. Degutis (1962) Comparison of skeletal ages and various physical and motor factors with the pubescent development of 10, 13, and 16 year old boys. *Res. Quart.* 33:356-368.

_____, and J. C. E. Harrison (1962) Differences in physical and motor traits between boys of advanced, normal, and retarded maturity. *Res. Quart.,* 33:13-25.

_____, R. N. Irving, and B. H. Heath (1961) Relation of maturity, structural, and strength measures to the somatotypes of boys 9 through 15 years of age. *Res. Quart.* 32:449-460.

_____ and K. H. Petersen (1961) Contrast of maturational, structural, and strength characteristics of athletes and nonathletes 10 to 15 years of age. *Res. Quart.,* 32:163-176.

_____, C. T. Shay, and D. K. Mathews (1955) Strength decrements from carrying various army packs on military marches. *Res. Quart.,* 26:253-265.

Clarke, M. F., and A. H. Smith (1938) Recovery following suppression of growth in the rat. *J. Nutr.,* 15:245-256.

Clayton, I. A. (1936) A study of the evidence of motor age based on technique of standing broad jump. Unpublished master's thesis, University of Wisconsin, Madison.

Coghill, G. E. (1929) *Anatomy and the Problem of Behaviour.* New York: Macmillan.

_____, and W. K. Legner (1937) Embryonic motility and sensitivity. (Trans. of Preyer, W., *Specielle Physiologie des Embryo.*) *Monogr. Soc. Res. Child Develpm.,* 2:1-115.

Comfort, Alex (1964) *Ageing, The Biology of Senescence*. New York: Holt, Rinehart and Winston, Inc.

Conel, J. L. (1939) *The Postnatal Development of the Human Cerebral Cortex. Vol. I. The Cortex of the Newborn*. Cambridge: Harvard University Press.

_____ (1941) *The Postnatal Development of the Human Cerebral Cortex. Vol. II. The Cortex of the One-month Infant*. Cambridge: Harvard University Press.

Cooley, D. G. (1963) Medicines of tomorrow. *Today's Health*, November: 38-42.

Corbin, K. B. and E. D. Gardner (1937) Decrease in number of myelinated fibers in human spinal roots with age. *Anat. Rec.*, 68:63-74.

Corey, E. L. (1931) Causative factors of the initial inspiration of the mammalian fetus. *Anat. Rec.*, 48(Suppl.):41.

Coronios, J. D. (1933) Development of behavior in the fetal cat. *Genet. Psychol. Monogr.* 14:283-386.

Cowan, E., and B. Pratt (1934) The hurdle jump as a developmental and diagnostic test. *Child Develpm.*, 5:107-121.

Cullumbine, H. (1949) Oral, rectal and axillary temperatures of adult Ceylonese. *Ceylon J. med. Sci. D.*, 6:88-90.

Cumbee, F. Z. (1954) A factorial analysis of motor co-ordination. *Res. Quart.* 25(4):412-428.

_____, M. Meyer, and G. Peterson (1957) Factorial analysis of motor coordination variables for third and fourth grade girls. *Res. Quart.*, 28:100-108.

Danzinger, L., and L. Frankl (1934) Zum Problem der Funktionsreifung. *Z. Kinderforsch.*, 43:219-254.

Dawson, P. M., and F. A. Hellebrandt (1945) The influence of aging in man upon his capacity for physical work and upon his cardio-vascular response to exercise. *Amer. J. Physiol.*, 143:420-427.

Deach, D. F. (1951) Genetic development of motor skills in children two through six years of age. *Microfilm Abstracts*, 11:287.

Dennis, W. (1934) A description and classification of the responses of the newborn infant. *Psychol. Bull.*, 31:5-22.

_____ (1935) The effect of restricted practice upon the reaching, sitting and standing of two infants. *J. Genet. Psychol.*, 47:17-32.

_____ (1938) Infant development under conditions of restricted practice and of minimum social stimulation: A preliminary report. *J. Genet. Psychol.*, 53:149-158.

_____ (1940) Does culture appreciably affect patterns of infant behavior? *J. Soc. Psychol.*, 12:305-317.

_____ (1941) Spalding's experiment on the flight of birds repeated with another species. *J. Comp. Psychol.*, 31:337-348.

_____, and M. G. Dennis (1940) The effect of cradling practices on the age of walking in Hopi children. *J. Genet. Psychol.,* 56:77-86.

Desroches, H. F., and B. D. Kaiman (1964) Stability of activity participation in an aged population. *J. Gerontol.* 19(2):211-214.

Deupree, R. H., and J. R. Simon (1963) Reaction time and movement time as a function of age, stimulus duration, and task difficulty. *Ergonomics,* 6(4):403-411.

Diettert, G. A. (1963) Circulation time in the aged. *J. Amer. Med. Assoc.,* 183(12):1037-1038.

Dill, D. B. (1942) Effects of physical strain and high altitudes on the heart and circulation. *Amer. Heart J.,* 23:441-454.

_____, A. Graybiel, A. Hurtado, and A. C. Taquini (1963) Gaseous exchange in the lungs in old age. *J. Amer. Geriat. Soc.,* 11(11):1063-1076.

_____, S. M. Horvath, and F. N. Craig (1958) Responses to exercise as related to age. *J. appl. Physiol.,* 12:195-196.

Dimock, H. S. (1935) A research in adolescence. I. Pubescence and physical growth. *Child Develpm.,* 6:177-195.

Dockeray, F. C., and C. Rice (1934) Responses of newborn infants to pain stimulation. *Ohio State Univ. Stud., Contrib. Psychol.,* 12:82-93.

Douday, D., and J. Tremolières (1947) Persistances d'importants déficits de croissance chez les enfants d'age scolaire en 1945-46. *Pr. med.,* 55:599-600.

Downing, M. E. (1947) Blood pressure of normal girls from three to sixteen years of age. *Amer. J. Dis. Child.,* 73-293-316.

Dublin, L. I., A. J. Lotka, and M. Spiegelman (1949) *Length of Life.* New York: The Ronald Press Company.

Dupertuis, C. W., and J. A. Hadden (1951) On the reconstruction of stature from long bones. *Amer. J. phys. Anthrop.,* 9:15-54.

_____, and N. B. Michael (1953). Comparison of growth in height and weight between ectomorphic and mesomorphic boys. *Child Develpm.,* 24:203-214.

Eccles, J. (1965) The synapse. *Sci. Amer.* 212(1):56-66.

Eckert, H. M. (1964) Linear relationships of isometric strength to propulsive force, angular velocity, and angular acceleration in the standing broad jump. *Res. Quart.* 35:298-306.

_____ (1965) A concept of force-energy in human movement. *J. Amer. Phys. Therapy Assoc.,* 45:213-218.

_____ and J. Day. Relationship between strength and work load in push-ups. Unpublished paper.

Edge, J. R., F. J. C. Millard, L. Reid, M. C. Path, and G. Simon (1964) The radiographic appearances of the chest in persons of advanced age. *Brit. J. Radiol.,* 37(442):769-774.

Ellis, R. W. B. (1945) Growth and health of Belgian children during and after the German occupation, 1940-1944. *Arch. Dis. Childh.*, 20:97-109.
_____ (1950) Age of puberty in the tropics. *Brit. med. J.*, 1:85-89.

Engle, E. T., R. E. Crafts, and C. E. Zeithaml (1937) First estrus in rats in relation to age, weight and length. *Proc. Soc. exp. Biol. (N.Y.)*, 37:427-432.

Espenschade, A. S. (1940) Motor performance in adolescence including the study of relationships with measures of physical growth and maturity. *Monogr. Soc. Res. Child Develpm.*, 5(1):1-126.
_____ (1947) Development of motor coordination in boys and girls. *Res. quart.*, 18:30-43.
_____ (1960) Motor development. In W. R. Johnson, (ed.), *Science and Medicine of Exercise and Sports.* New York: Harper & Row, Publishers.
_____ (1963) Restudy of relationships between physical performances of school children and age, height, and weight. *Res. Quart.*, 34(2):144-153.
_____, R. R. Dable, and R. Schoendube (1953) Dynamic balance in adolescent boys. *Res. Quart.*, 24:270-275.
_____ and H. E. Meleney (1961) Motor performances of adolescent boys and girls of today in comparison with those of 24 years ago. *Res. Quart.*, 32:186-189.

Feldman, W. M. (1920) *Principles of Antenatal and Postnatal Child Psychology, Pure and Applied.* New York: Longmans, Green & Co.

Ferris, B. G., and C. W. Smith (1953) Maximum breathing capacity and vital capacity in female children and adolescents. *Pediatrics*, 12:341-252.
_____, J. L. Whittenberger, and J. R. Gallagher (1952) Maximum breathing capacity and vital capacity of male children and adolescents. *Pediatrics*, 9:659-670.

Fitzgerald, J. E., and W. F. Windle (1942) Some observations on early human fetal movements. *J. Comp. Neurol.*, 76:159-167.

Froeschels, E., and H. Beebe (1946) Testing the hearing of newborn infants. *Arch. Otolaryng.*, 44:710-714.

Garn, S. M. (1960) Fat accumulation and aging in males and females. In B. L. Strehler, (ed.) *The Biology of Aging.* Washington, D.C. American Institute of Biological Sciences.
_____, and L. C. Clark (1953) The sex difference in the basal metabolic rate. *Child Develpm.*, 24:215-224.
_____, and _____, and R. Portray (1953) Relationship between body composition and basal metabolic rate in children. *J. appl. Physiol.*, 6:163-167.

Gates, A. I. (1924) The nature and educational significance of physical status and of mental, physiological, social and emotional maturity. *J. Educ. Psychol.,* 15.329-358.

Gesell, A. (1928) *Infancy and Human Growth.* New York: Macmillan & Co.

―――― (1933) Maturation and the patterning of behavior. In C. Murchison (ed.), *A Handbook of Child Psychology.* Worcester: Clark University Press. Second Edition.

―――― (1954) The ontogenesis of infant behavior. In L. Carmichael, (ed.), *Manual of Child Psychology.* New York: John Wiley & Sons, Inc., Second Edition.

――――, and L. B. Ames (1940) The ontogenetic organization of prone behavior in human infancy. *J. Genet. Psychol.,* 56:247-263.

――――, and ―――― (1947) The development of handedness. *J. Genet. Psychol.,* 70:155-175.

――――, and F. L. Ilg (1937) *The Feeding Behavior of Infants: A Pediatric Approach to the Mental Hygiene of Early Life.* Philadelphia: J. B. Lippincott Co.

――――, and ―――― (1946) *The Child from Five to Ten.* New York: Harper & Row, Publishers.

――――, and H. Thompson (1929) Learning and growth in identical infant twins: An experimental study of the method of co-twin control. *Genet. Psychol. Monogr.,* 6:1-124.

――――, and ―――― (1934) *Infant Behavior: Its Genesis and Growth.* New York: McGraw-Hill.

――――, and ―――― (1938) *The Psychology of Early Growth.* New York: Macmillan & Co.

Glassow, R. B., and P. Kruse (1960) Motor performance of girls age 6 to 14 years. *Res. Quart.,* 31(3):426-433.

Goetzinger, C. P. (1961) A reevaluation of the Heath railwalking test. *J. Educ. Res.* 54:187-191.

Golding, L. A. (1961) The effects of physical training upon total serum cholesterol levels. *Res. Quart.* 32(4):499-506.

Goodenough, F. L. (1945) *Developmental Psychology: An Introduction to the Study of Human Behavior.* New York: Appleton-Century.

Goss, C. M. (1940) First contractions of the heart without cytological differentiation. *Anat. Rec.,* 76:19-27.

Graux, P., G. C. Guazzi, and C. Gesquiere (1962) Spinal cord of the aged. *Rev. Neurol.,* 107(4):337-352.

Guttridge, M. V. (1939) A study of motor achievements of young children. *Arch. Psychol.,* 244:1-178.

Hale, Creighton J. (1956) Physiological maturity of Little League Baseball players. *Res. Quart.,* 27:276-284.

Halverson, H. M. (1931) An experimental study of prehension in infants by means of systematic cinema records., *Gent. Psychol. Monogr.*, 10:107-286.

_____ (1937) Studies of the grasping responses of early infancy: I, II, III. *J. Genet. Psychol.*, 51:371-449.

_____ (1940) Genital and sphincter behavior of the male infant. *J. Genet. Psychol.*, 56:95-136.

_____ (1941) Variations in pulse and respiration during different phases of infant behavior. *J. Genet. Psychol.*, 59:259-330.

_____ (1944) Mechanisms of early infant feeding. *J. Genet. Psychol.*, 64:185-223.

Halverson, L. E., and M. A. Roberton (1966) A Study of motor pattern development in young children. Report at National Convention, American Association for Health, Physical Education and Recreation.

Harrison, R. G. (1914) The reaction of embryonic cells to solid surfaces. *J. exp. Zool.*, 17:521-544.

Harrison, Virginia F. (1962) Review of the neuromuscular bases for motor learning. *Res. Quart.*, 33:59-69.

Hartman, C. G. (1936) *Time of Ovulation in Women*. Baltimore: Williams and Wilkins.

Hartman, D. M. (1943) The hurdle jump as a measure of the motor proficiency of young children. *Child Develpm.*, 14:201-211.

Havighurst, R. J. (1950) *Developmental Tasks and Education*. New York: Longmans, Green.

Heath, S. R. (1949) The rail walking test: Preliminary maturational norms for boys and girls. *Motor Skills Res. Exchg.*, 1:34-36.

Hejinian, L., and E. Hatt (1929) The stem-length:recumbent-length as an index of body type in young children. *Amer. J. Phys. Anthrop.*, 13:287-307.

Hellebrandt, F. A., G. L. Rarick, R. Glassow, and M. L. Carns (1961) Physiological analysis of basic motor skills. I. Growth and development of jumping. *Amer. J. Phys. Med.*, 40:14-25.

Hess, J. H. (1922) *Premature and Congenitally Diseased Infants*. Philadelphia: Lea and Febiger.

Heyman, D. K., and F. C. Jeffers (1964) Study of the relative influence of race and socio-economic status upon the activities and attitudes of a southern aged population. *J. Gerontol.*, 19(2):225-229.

Hicks, C. B. (1963) Why are twins so special? *Today's Health*. December: 18-21, 72-76.

Hildreth, G. (1948) Manual dominance in nursery school children. *J. Genet. Psychol.*, 73:29-45.

_____ (1949) The development and training of hand dominance: I.

Characteristics of handedness; II. Developmental tendencies in handedness; III. Origin of handedness and lateral dominance. *J. Genet. Psychol.*, 75:197-275.

———— (1950) The development and training of hand dominance; IV. Developmental problems associated with handedness; V. Training of handedness. *J. Genet. Psychol.*, 76:39-144.

Hilgard, J. R. (1932) Learning and maturation in preschool children. *J. Genet. Psychol.*, 41:36-56.

Hinchcliffe, R. (1962) Aging and sensory thresholds. *J. Gerontol.*, 17 (1):45-50.

Hogg, I. D. (1941) Sensory nerves and associated structures in the skin of human fetuses of 8 to 14 weeks of menstrual age correlated with functional capability. *J. Comp. Neurol.*, 75:371-410.

Hooker, D. (1939) Fetal behavior. *Res. Publ. Ass. Nerv. Ment. Dis.*, 19:237-243.

———— (1944) *The Origin of Overt Behavior.* Ann Arbor: University of Michigan Press.

Horrocks, J. E. (1954) The adolescent. In L. Carmichael, (ed.), *Manual of Child Psychology.* New York: John Wiley & Sons, Inc.

Howe, P. E., and M. Schiller (1952) Growth responses of the school child to changes in diet and environmental factors. *J. appl. Physiol.*, 5:51-61.

Huggett, A. S. G. (1930) Foetal respiratory reflexes. *J. Physiol.*, 69:144-152.

Hughes, J. G., B. Ehemann, and W. A. Brown (1948) Electroencephalography of the newborn. III. Brain potentials of babies born of mothers given seconal sodium. *Amer. J. Dis. Child.*, 76:626-633.

Hunsicker, P. A. and G. G. Reiff (1966) A survey and comparison of youth fitness 1958-1965. *J. Health P.E Rec.* 37:23-25.

Hupprich, F. L., and P. O. Sigerseth (1950) The specificity of flexibility in girls. *Res. Quart.*, 21:25-33.

Hurdle, A. D. F., and A. J. Rosin (1962) Red cell volume and red cell survival in normal aged people. *J. Clin. Pathol.*, 15(4):343-345.

Hurlock, Elizabeth B. (1953) *Developmental Psychology.* New York: McGraw-Hill Book Co., Inc.

Hurme, V. O. (1949) Ranges of normalcy in the eruption of the permanent teeth. *J. Dent. Child.*, 16:11-15.

Iliff, A., and V. A. Lee (1952) Pulse rate, respiratory rate, and body temperature of children between two months and eighteen years of age. *Child Develpm.*, 23:237-245.

Irwin, O. C. (1932) The distribution of the amount of motility in young infants between two nursing periods. *J. Comp. Psychol.*, 14:429-445.

———— (1936) Qualitative changes in a vertebral reaction pattern during infancy: A motion picture study. *Univ. Iowa Stud. Child Welfare*, 12:201-207.

_____ (1941) Effect of strong light on the body activity of newborns. *J. Comp. Psychol.*, 32:233-236.

_____ (1942) Can infants have IQ's? *Psychol. Rev.*, 49:69-79.

_____, and A. P. Weiss (1930) A note on mass activity in newborn infants. *J. Genet. Psychol.*, 38:20-30.

_____, and L. A. Weiss (1934) The effect of clothing on the general and vocal activity of the newborn infant. *Univ. Iowa Stud. Child Welfare*, 9:149-162.

Ito, P. K. (1942) Comparative biometrical study of physique of Japanese. women born and reared under different environments. *Hum. Biol.*, 14:279-351.

Jackson, C. M. (1928) Some aspects of form and growth. In W. J. Robbins, S. Brody, A. G. Hogan, C. M. Jackson, and C. W. Green, *Growth*. New Haven: Yale University Press.

Jenkins, L. M. (1930) *A Comparative Study of Motor Achievements of Children Five, Six and Seven Years of Age.* New York: Teachers College, Columbia University.

Jensen, K. (1932) Differential reactions to taste and temperature stimuli in newborn infants. *Genet. Psychol. Monogr.*, 12:363-479.

Jersild, A. T., and R. Tasch (1949) *Children's Interests and What They Suggest for Education.* New York: Bureau of Publications, Teachers College, Columbia University.

Johnson, B. (1925) *Mental Growth of Children in Relation to the Rate of Growth in Bodily Development: A Report of the Bureau of Educational Experiments.* New York: Dutton.

Johnson, M. W. (1935) The effect on behavior of variation in the amount of play equipment. *Child Develpm.*, 6:56-68.

Jokl, E. (1954) *Alter und Leistung.* Berlin: Springer Verlag.

Jones, H. E. (1949) *Motor Performance and Growth.* Berkeley: University of California Press.

_____, and M. C. Jones (1957) *Adolescence.* Berkeley: University Extension, University of California.

Jones, T. D. (1939) The development of certain motor skills and play activities in young children. *Child Develpm. Monogr. Teachers College, Columbia University*, No. 26:1-180.

Kane, R. J., and H. V. Meredith (1952) Ability in the standing broad jump of school children 7, 9 and 11 years of age. *Res. Quart.*, 23:198-208.

Kawin, E. (1934) *The Wise Choice of Toys.* Chicago: University of Chicago Press.

Kemsley, W. F. F. (1953) Changes in body weight from 1943 to 1950. *Ann. Eugen., Lond.*, 18:22-42.

Keogh, Jack (1965) *Motor Performance of Elementary School Children.* Los Angeles: Department of Physical Education, University of California.

Kiil, V. (1939) Stature and growth of Norwegian men during the past 200 years. *Skr. norske Vidensk Akad.*, No. 6.

Kohn, R. R., and E. Rollerson (1959) Age changes in swelling properties of human myocardium. *Proc. Soc. Exp. Biol., N.Y.*, 100:253-256.

Krogman, W. M. (1948) A handbook of the measurement and interrelation of height and weight in the growing child. *Monogr. Soc. Res. Child Develpm.*, 13(3).

———— (1950) The concept of maturity from a morphological viewpoint. *Child Develpm.*, 21:25-32.

———— (1959) Maturation age of 55 boys in the Little League World Series, 1957. *Res. Quart.*, 30:54-56.

Landis, C., and W. A. Hunt. (1939) *The Startle Pattern.* New York: Farrar and Rinehart.

Landiss, Carl W. (1955) Influences of physical education activities on motor ability and physical fitness of male freshmen. *Res. Quart.*, 26(3):295-307.

Landreth, C. (1958) *The Psychology of Early Childhood.* New York: Alfred A. Knopf.

Langley, J., and H. Anderson (1904) The union of different kinds of nerve fibers. *J. Physiol.*, 31:365-391.

Langworthy, O. R. (1933) Development of behavior patterns and myelinization of the nervous system in the human fetus and infant. *Contr. Embryol. Carn. Instn.*, 24:1-57.

Lansing, A. I. (1959) General biology of senescence. In J. E. Birren (ed.), *Handbook of Aging and the Individual.* Chicago: The University of Chicago Press.

Larson, L. A. (1946) Some findings resulting from the Army Air Forces Physical Training Program. *Res. Quart.*, 17:144-164.

Lehman, Harvey C. (1953) *Age and Achievement.* Published for the American Philosophical Society by Princeton University Press, Princeton, N.J.

Lewis, R. C., A. M. Duval, and A. Iliff (1943) Standards for the basal metabolism of children from 2 to 15 years of age, inclusive. *J. Pediat.*, 23:1-18.

Ley, L. (1938) Über die Menarche der Frau und ihre Beziehungen zur Pigmentation: Untersuchungen am Schulkindern der Stadt Mainz. *Arch. Gynak.*, 165:489-503.

Liddell, E. G. T., and C. S. Sherrington (1925) Recruitment and some other features of reflex inhibition. *Proc. Roy. Soc.; Series B. Biol. Sci.*, 97:488-518.

Ling, B. C. (1942) I. A genetic study of sustained visual fixation and associated behavior in the human infant from birth to six months. *J. Genet. Psychol.*, 61:227-277.

Lippman, H. S. (1927) Certain behavior responses in early infancy. *J. Genet. Psychol.*, 34:424-440.

Lloyd, D. P. C. (1946) Principles of spinal reflex activity. In J. F. Fulton, (ed.), *Howell's Textbook of Physiology.* Philadelphia: Saunders.

Lombard, O. M. (1950) Breadth of bone and muscle by age and sex in childhood. *Child Develpm.*, 21:229-239.

McCarthy, D. A. (1930) *The Language Development of the Preschool Child.* Minneapolis: University of Minnesota Press.

McCaskill, C. L., and B. L. Wellman (1938) A study of common motor achievements at the preschool ages. *Child Develpm.*, 9:141-150.

McCloy, C. H. (1936) Appraising physical status: The selection of measurements. *Univ. Iowa Stud. Child Welfare.*, 12(2):1-126.

_____ (1945) *Tests and Measurements in Health and Physical Education.* New York: Crofts.

McFarland, R. A., G. S. Tune, and A. T. Welford (1964) On the driving of automobiles by older people. *J. Gerontol.*, 19(2):190-197.

McGinnis, J. M. (1930) Eye-movements and optic nystagmus in early infancy. *Genet. Psychol. Monogr.*, 8:321-430.

McGraw, M. B. (1935) *Growth: A Study of Johnny and Jimmy.* New York: Appleton-Century.

_____ (1939a) Behavior of the newborn infant and early neuromuscular development. *Res. Publ. Ass. Nerv. Ment. Dis.*, 19:244-246.

_____ (1939b) Later development of children specially trained during infancy. *Child Develpm.*, 10:1-19.

_____ (1940a) Neuromuscular development of the human infant as exemplified in the achievement of erect locomotion. *J. Pediat.*, 17:747-771.

_____ (1940b) Neuromuscular mechanism of the infant. Development reflected by postural adjustments to an inverted position. *Amer. J. Dis. Child.*, 60:1031-1042.

_____ (1941a) Development of neuro-muscular mechanisms as reflected in the crawling and creeping behavior of the human infant. *J. Genet. Psychol.*, 58:83-111.

_____ (1941b) Development of rotary-vestibular reactions of the human infant. *Child Develpm*, 12:17-19.

_____ (1946) Maturation of behavior. In L. Carmichael (ed.), *Manual of Child Psychology.* New York: John Wiley & Sons, Inc.

McKusick, V. A. (1965) The royal hemophelia. *Sci. Amer.*, 213(2):88-95.

Mangarov, I. (1964) Physical development and capacity of Bulgarian students. *Bulletin d'Information, Bulgarian Olympic Com.,* Year IX, No. 5.

Maresh, H. M. (1943) Growth of major long bones in healthy children. A preliminary report on successive roentgenograms of the extremities from early infancy to twelve years of age. *Amer. J. Dis. Child.,* 66:227-257.

Marloff, H. J. (1949) Werte des erythrocitären Systems bei 40 jungen Sport-treibenden Frauen. *Pflüg. Arch. ges. Physiol.,* 251:241-254.

Martin, E. G. (1918) Muscular strength and muscular symmetry in human beings. *Amer. J. Physiol.,* 46:67-83.

Master, A. M. (1935) The two-step test of myocardial function. *Amer. Heart J.,* 10(4):495-510.

Mayer, R. F. (1963) Nerve conduction studies in man. *Neurology,* 13(12): 1021-1030.

Mead, M. (1930) *Growing up in New Guinea.* New York: William Morrow & Co.

Meredith, H. V. (1935) The rhythm of physical growth: A study of 18 anthropometric measures on Iowa City males ranging in age between birth and 18 years. *Univ. Iowa Stud. Child Welfare,* 11(3).

_____ (1946) Order and age of eruption for the deciduous dentition. *J. dent. Res.,* 25:43-66.

_____, and B. Boynton (1937) The transverse growth of the extremities: An analysis of girth measurements for arm, forearm, thigh and leg taken on Iowa City white children. *Hum. Biol.,* 9:366-403.

Metheny, E. (1941a) Breathing capacity and grip strength of preschool children. *Univ. Iowa Stud. Child Welfare.,* 18(2):1-207.

_____ (1941b) The present status of strength testing for children of elementary school and preschool age. *Res Quart.,* 12:115-130.

Meyer, M. H. (1951) A longitudinal study of certain motor activities of elementary school children. Unpublished study, University of Wisconsin, Madison.

Michael, E. D., and A. Gallon (1959) Periodic changes in the circulation during athletic training as reflected by a step test. *Res. Quart.,* 30(3):303-311.

Michelson, N. (1944) Studies in physical development of Negroes. IV. Onset of puberty. *Amer. J. phys. Anthrop.,* 2:151-166.

Miles, W. R. (1950) Simultaneous right- and left-hand grip. Vol. 3. In R. W. Gerard (ed.), *Methods in Medical Research.* Chicago: Year Book Publishers.

Mills, C. A. (1949) Temperature dominance over human life. *Science,* 110:267-271.

_____ (1950) Temperature influence over human growth and development. *Hum. Biol.*, 22:71-74.

Minkowski, M. (1921) Ueber Bewegungen und Reflexe des menschlichen Foetus während der ersten Hälfte seiner Entwicklung. *Schweiz. Arch. Neurol. Psychiat.*, 8:148-151.

_____ (1922) Ueber frühzeitige Bewegungen. Reflexe und muskuläre Reaktionen beim menschlichen Fötus und ihre Beziehungen zum fötalen Nerven- und Muskelsystem. *Schweiz. med. Wschr.*, 52:721-724.

_____ (1924) Zum gengenwärtigen Stand der Lehre von den Reflexen in entwicklungsgeschichtlicher und der anatomischphysiologischer Beziehung. *Schweiz. Arch. Neurol. Psychiat.*, 15:239-259.

_____ (1926) Sur les modalités et la localisation du réflexe plantaire au cours de son évolution du foetus à l'adulte. *C. R. Congr. Medecins. Alienistes et Neurologistes de France, Geneva,* 30:301-308.

_____ (1928) Neurobiologische Studien am menschenlichen Foetus. *Handb. Biol. ArbMeth.*, 5B:511-618.

Minot, C. S. (1892) *Human Embryology*. New York: William Wood.

Montoye, Henry J., W. D. Van Huss, H. W. Olson, W. R. Pierson, and A. J. Hudec (1957) *The Longevity and Morbidity of College Athletes*. Phi Epsilon Kappa Fraternity.

Morris, C. B. (1948) The measurement of the strength of muscle relative to the cross-section. *Res. Quart.*, 19:295-303.

Morris, J. N., J. A. Heady, P. A. B. Raffle, C. G. Roberts and J. W. Parks (1953) Coronary heart disease and physical activity of work. *Lancet,* 265:1053-1057.

Morse, M., F. W. Schultz, and D. E. Cassels (1952) The lung volume and its subdivisions in boys 10—17 years of age. *J. Clin. Invest.*, 31:380-391.

Mugrage, E. R., and M. I. Andresen (1936) Values for red blood cells of average infants and children. *Amer. J. Dis. Child.*, 51:775-791.

_____, and _____ (1938) Red blood cell values in adolescence. *Amer. J. Dis. Child.*, 56:997-1003.

National Foundation—March of Dimes (Pamphlet) With best wishes for a happy birthday from the National Foundation.

Needham, J. (1931) *Chemical Embryology*. Cambridge: University Press.

Neilson, N. P., and F. W. Cozens (1934) *Achievement Scales in Physical Education Activities*. Sacramento: State Dept. of Education.

Nelson, M. M., C. W. Asling, and H. M. Evans (1952) Production of multiple congenital abnormalities in young by pteroylglutamic acid deficiency during gestation. *J. Nutrition,* 48:61-80.

Nelson, R. C., and R. A. Fahrney (1965) Relationship between strength and speed of elbow flexion. *Res. Quart.*, 36:455-463.

Nevers, J. E. (1948) The effects of physiological age on motor achievement. *Res. Quart.*, 19:103-110.

Newbery, H. (1941) Studies in fetal behavior. IV. The measurement of three types of fetal activity. *J. Comp. Psychol.*, 32:521-530.

Nicolson, A. B., and C. Hanley (1953) Indices of physiological maturity: Derivation and inter-relationships. *Child Develpm.*, 24:3-38.

Norman, J. R., I. H. Schweppe, E. Salazar, and J. H. Knowles (1964) Lung changes and aging: A review of a report of changes in 43 Spanish-American War Veterans. *J. Amer. Geriat. Soc.*, 12(1):38-49.

Norris, A. H., and N. W. Shock (1960) Exercise in the adult years—with special reference to the advanced years. In W. R. Johnson, (ed.), *Science and Medicine of Exercise and Sports.* New York: Harper.

_____ and _____, and M. J. Yiengst (1953) Age changes in heart rate and blood pressure responses to tilting and standardized exercise. *Circulation*, 8:521-526.

Norval, M. A. (1947) Relationship of weight and length of infants at birth to the age at which they begin to walk alone. *J. Pediat.*, 30:676-678.

Nylin, G. (1935) The physiology of the circulation during puberty. *Acta med. scand.*, 69(Suppl.).

Olmsted, J. M. D. (1931) The nerve as a formative influence in the development of taste-buds. *J. comp. Neurol.*, 31:465-468.

Palmer, C. E. (1933) Seasonal variations of average growth in weight of elementary school children. *Pbl. Hlth. Rep., Wash.*, 48:211-233.

Peiper, A. (1926) Ueber die Helligkeits und Farbenempfindungen der Fruhgeburten. *Arch Kinderheilk.*, 80:1-20.

_____ (1939) Die Führung des Saugzentrums durch das Schluckzentrum. *Pflüg. Arch. ges. Physiol.*, 242:751-755.

_____ (1951) Die Schnappatmung in Filmausschnitten. *Kinderarztliche Praxis*, 19:272-279.

Piatt, J. (1940) Nerve-muscle specificity in Amblystoma, studied by means of heterotopic cord grafts. *J. Exp. Zool.*, 85:211-237.

_____ (1942) Transplantation of aneurogenic forelimbs in Amblystoma punctatum. *J. Exp. Zool.*, 91:79-101.

Pierson, I. M., and H. J. Montoye (1958) Movement time, reaction time, and age. *J. Gerontol.*, 13:418-421.

Pratt, K. C. (1930) Note on the relation of temperature and humidity on the activity of young infants. *J. Genet. Psychol.*, 38:480-484.

_____ (1954) The neonate. In L. Carmichael, (ed), *Manual of Child Psychology.* New York: John Wiley & Sons. Second Edition.

_____, A. K. Nelson, and K. H. Sun (1930) The behavior of the newborn infant. *Ohio State Univ. Stud. Contr. Psychol.*, No. 10.

Pressey, S. L., and R. G. Kuhlen (1957) *Psychological Development through the Life Span.* New York: Harper & Row, Publishers.

Pryor, H. B. (1936) Certain physical and physiological aspects of adolescent development in girls. *J. Pediat.,* 8:52-62.

————, and H. R. Stolz (1933) Determining appropriate weight for body build. *J. Pediat.,* 3:608-622.

Rarick, G. L. (1954) *Motor Development during Infancy and Childhood.* Mimeographed monograph. Madison, Wis.: University of Wisconsin.

————, and R. McKee (1949) A study of twenty third grade children exhibiting extreme levels of achievements on tests of motor proficiency. *Res. Quart.,* 20:142-150.

————, and Nancy Oyster (1964) Physical maturity, muscular strength, and motor performance of young school-age boys. *Res. Quart.,* 35:523-531.

————, and J. A. Thompson (1956) Roentenographic measures of leg muscle size and ankle extensor strength of seven-year-old children. *Res. Quart.,* 27:321-322.

Reilly, F. J. (1917) *New Rational Athletics for Boys and Girls.* Boston: Heath.

Reynolds, E. L. (1943) Degree of kinship and pattern of ossification. *Amer. J. phys. Anthrop.,* 1:405-416.

———— (1944) Differential tissue growth in the leg during childhood. *Child Develpm.,* 15:181-205.

———— (1945) The bony pelvic girdle in early infancy. *Amer. J. Phys. Anthrop.,* 3:321-354.

———— (1947) The bony pelvis in prepuberal childhood. *Amer. J. Phys. Anthrop.,* 5:165-200.

————, and G. Schoen (1947) Growth patterns of identical triplets from eight through eighteen years. *Child Develpm.,* 18:130-151.

————, and L. W. Sontag (1944) Seasonal variations in weight, height and appearance of ossification centers. *J. Pediat.,* 24:524-535.

————, and J. V. Wines (1948) Individual differences in physical changes associated with adolescence in girls. *Amer. J. Dis. Child.,* 75:329-350.

————, and ———— (1951) Physical changes associated with adolescence in boys. *Amer. J. Dis. Child.,* 82:529-547.

Richards, T. W., and O. C. Irwin (1934) Plantar responses of infants and young children: An examination of the literature and reports of new experiments. *Univ. Iowa Stud. Child Welfare,* No. 11.

————, H. Newbery, and R. Fallgatter (1938) Studies in fetal behavior. II. Activity of the human fetus *in utero* and its relation to other prenatal conditions, particularly the mother's basal metabolic rate. *Child Develpm.,* 9:69-78.

Richey, H. G. (1931) The blood pressure in boys and girls before and after puberty. Its relation to growth and to maturity. *Amer. J. Dis. Child.,* 42:1281-1330.

———— (1937) Relation of accelerated, normal and retarded puberty to the height and weight of school children. *Monog. Soc. Res. Child Develpm.,* 2(1):1-67.

Richter, C. P. (1934) The grasp reflex of the newborn infant. *Amer. J. Dis. Child.,* 48:327-332.

Robinow, M., T. W. Richards, and M. Anderson (1942) The eruption of deciduous teeth. *Growth,* 6:127-133.

Robinson, S. (1938) Experimental studies of physical fitness in relation to age. *Arb. Physiol.,* 10:251-323.

Rochelle, R. H. (1961) Blood plasma cholesterol changes during a physical training program. *Res. Quart.,* 32(4):538-550.

Romanes, G. J. (1947) The prenatal medullation of the sheep's nervous system. *J. Anat. Lond.,* 81:64-81.

Ruja, H. (1948) Relation between neonate crying and length of labor. *J. Genet. Psychol.,* 73:53-55.

Sager, Ruth (1965) Genes outside the chromosomes. *Sci. Amer.,* 212(1):71-79.

Saunders, J. W. (1947) The proximo-distal sequence of origin of wing parts and the role of the ectoderm. *Anat. Rec.,* 99:11.

Schaie, K. W., P. Baltes, and C. R. Strother (1964) A study of auditory sensitivity in advanced age. *J. Gerontol.,* 19(4):453-457.

Schaub, M. C. (1964/5) The aging of collagen in the heart muscle. *Gerontologia,* 10(1):38-41.

Scheinfeld, Amram (1939) *You and Heredity.* New York: Frederick A. Stokes Co.

Schmidt, L. (1950) Der "erste" Atemzug. *Mschr. Kinderheilk.,* 98:213-217.

Scott, R. B., W. W. Cardozo, A. DeG. Smith, and M. R. DeLilly (1950) Growth and development of Negro infants: III. Growth during the first year of life as observed in private pediatric practice. *J. Pediat.,* 37:885-893.

Seashore, H. G. (1947) The development of a beam walking test and its use in measuring development of balance in children. *Res. Quart.,* 18:246-259.

Seils, L. G. (1951) The relationship between measures of physical growth and gross motor performance of primary-grade school children. *Res. Quart.,* 22:244-260.

Sheldon, J. H. (1950) Medical-social aspects of the aging process. In M. Derber, (ed.), *The Aged and Society*. Champaign, Ill.: Industrial Relations Research Association.

———— (1963) The effect of age on the control of sway. *Gerontol. Clin. (Basel)*, 5(3):129-138.

Sheldon, W. H., S. S. Stevens, and W. B. Tucker (1940). *The Varieties of Human Physique*. New York: Harper & Row, Publishers.

Sherman, E. D., and E. Robillard (1964) Sensitivity to pain in relationship to age. *J. Amer. Geriat. Soc.*, 12(11):1037-1044.

Sherman, M., and I. C. Sherman (1925) Sensorimotor responses in infants. *J. Comp. Psychol.*, 5:53-68.

———— and ————, and C. D. Flory (1936) Infant behavior. *Comp. Psychol. Monogr.*, 12(4).

Shirley, M. M. (1931) *The First Two Years: A Study of Twenty-five Babies. Vol. I. Postural and Locomotor Development*. Minneapolis: University of Minnesota Press.

———— (1933) *The First Two Years: A Study of Twenty-five Babies. Vol. II. Intellectual Development*. Minneapolis: University of Minnesota Press.

Shock, N. W. (1941) Age changes and sex differences in alveolar CO_2 tension. *Amer. J. Physiol.*, 133:610-616.

———— (1944) Basal blood pressure and pulse rate in adolescents. *Amer. J. Dis. Child.*, 68:16-22.

———— (1946) Physiological responses of adolescents to exercise. *Texas Rep. Biol. Med.*, 4:368-386.

————, Editor. (1952) *Problems of Aging*. New York: Josiah Macy, Jr. Foundation.

————, Editor. (1960) *Aging . . . Some Social and Biological Aspects*. American Assoc. for the Advancement of Science, Washington, D.C.

———— (1962) The physiology of aging. *Sci. Amer.*, 206(1):100-110.

————, and M. H. Soley (1939) Average values for basal respiratory functions in adolescents and adults. *J. Nutr.*, 18:143-153.

Shuttleworth, F. K. (1939) The physical and mental growth of girls and boys age six to nineteen in relation to age at maximum growth. *Monogr. Soc. Res. Child Develpm.*, 4(3):1-291.

———— (1949) The adolescent period: a graphic atlas. *Monogr. Soc. Res. Child Develpm.*, 14, Serial No. 49, No. 1.

Simmons, K. (1944) The Brush Foundation study of child growth and development. II. Physical growth and development. *Mongr. Soc. Res. Child Develpm.*, 9(1):1-87.

————, and T. W. Todd (1938) Growth of well children: Analysis of stature and weight, 3 months to 13 years. *Growth*, 2:93-143.

Simonson, E. (1957) Changes in physical fitness and cardiovascular functions with age. *Geriatrics,* 12:28-39.

_____, W. M. Kearns, and N. Enzer (1941) Effect of oral administration of methyltestosterone on fatigue in eunuchoids and castrates. *Endocrinology,* 28:506-512.

Sjöstrand, T. (1953) Volume and distribution of blood and their significance in regulating the circulation. *Physiol. Rev.,* 33:202-228.

Sloan, A. W. (1963) Physical fitness of college students in South Africa, United States of America, and England. *Res. Quart.,* 34(2):244-248.

Sontag, L. W., and R. F. Wallace (1936) Changes in the rate of the human fetal heart in response to vibratory stimuli. *Amer. J. Dis. Child.,* 51:583-589.

Spalding, D. A. (1873) Instinct; with original observations on young animals. *Macmillan's Mag.,* 27:282-293.

_____ (1875) Instinct and acquisition. *Nature,* 12:507-508.

Speidel, C. C. (1946) Prolonged histories of vagus nerve regeneration patterns, sterile distal stumps and sheath cell outgrowths. *Anat. Rec.,* 94:55.

_____ (1948) Correlated studies of sense organs and nerves of the lateral-line in living frog tadpoles. II. The trophic influence of specific nerve supply as revealed by prolonged observations of denervated and re-innervated organs. *Amer. J. Anat.,* 82:277-320.

Spelt, D. K. (1948) The conditioning of the human fetus *in utero. J. Exp. Psychol.,* 38:338-346.

Sperry, R. W. (1942) Reestablishment of visuomotor coordinations by optic nerve regeneration. *Anat. Rec.,* 84:470.

_____ (1943) Visuomotor coordination in the newt *(Triturus viridescens)* after regeneration of the optic nerve. *J. comp. Neurol.,* 79:33-55.

_____ (1944) Optic nerve regeneration with return of vision in anurans. *J. Neurophysiol.,* 7:57-69.

_____ (1951) Mechanisms of neural maturation. In S. S. Stevens, (ed.), *Handbook of Experimental Psychology.* New York: John Wiley & Sons, Inc.

Spiegelman, M. (1960) Factors in human mortality. In B. L. Strehler, (ed.) *The Biology of Aging.* Washington, D.C.: American Institute of Biological Sciences.

Stirnimann, F. (1939) Versuche über die Reaktionen Neugeborener auf Wärme- und Kältereize. *Z. Kinderpsychiat.,* 5:143-150.

_____ (1944) Ueber das Farbempfinden Neugeborener. *Ann. Paediat.,* 163:1-25.

Stolz, H. R., and L. M. Stolz (1951) *Somatic Development of Adolescent Boys. A Study of the Growth of Boys during the Second Decade of Life.* New York: Macmillan.

Strandell, T. (1964) Heart rate and work load at minimal working intensity in old men. *Acta Med. Scand.,* 176(3):301-318.

Streeter, G. L. (1920) Weight, sitting height, head size, foot length, and menstrual age of the human embryo. *Contr. Embryol., Carnegie Inst. Wash.,* 11(55):143-170.

Strehler, Bernard L., Editor. (1960) *The Biology of Aging.* Washington, D.C., American Institute of Biological Sciences.

Strong, E. K. (1931) *Changes of Interest with Age.* Stanford, Calif.: Stanford University Press.

Stubbs, E. M. (1934) The effect of the factors of duration, intensity, and and pitch of sound stimuli on the responses of newborn infants. *Univ. Iowa Stud. Child Welfare,* 9(4):75-135.

————, and O. C. Irwin (1933) Laterality of limb movements of four newborn infants. *Child Develpm.,* 4:358-359.

Sullivan, F. J., A. D. Bender, and S. M. Horvath (1963) The aging cell. *J. Amer. Geriat. Soc.,* 11(10):923-932.

Tanner, J.M. (1951) The relationships between the frequency of the heart, oral temperature and rectal temperature in man at rest. *J. Physiol.,* 115:391-409.

———— (1955) *Growth at Adolescence.* Oxford: Blackwell Scientific Publications.

Taylor, R. (1917) Hunger in the infant. *Amer. J. Dis. Child.,* 14:233-257.

Terman, L. M., and M. A. Merrill (1937) *Measuring Intelligence.* New York: Houghton Mifflin & Co.

Tisserand-Perrier, M. (1953) Etude comparative de certains processus de croissance chez les jumeaux. *J. Génét. Hum.,* 2:87-102.

Thompson, Helen (1954) Physical growth. In L. Carmichael, (ed.) , *Manual of Child Psychology.* New York: John Wiley & Sons, Inc.

Updegraff, R. (1932) Preferential handedness in young children. *J. Exp. Educ.,* 1:134-139.

Valentine, W. L., and I. Wagner (1934) Relative arm motility in the newborn infant. *Ohio State Univ. Stud.,* 12:53-68.

Van Alstyne, D. (1932) *Play Behavior and Choice of Play Materials of Preschool Children.* Chicago: University of Chicago Press.

Verhaegen, P. and A. Ntumba (1964) Note on the frequency of left-handedness in African children. *J. Educ. Psychol.,* 55:89-90.

Verzár, F. (1963) The aging of collagen. *Sci. Amer.* 208(4):104-114.

Victors, E. E. (1961) A cinematographical analysis of catching behavior of a selected group of seven and nine year old boys. *Dissert. Abstracts,* 22:1903-1904.

von Mering, O., and F. L. Weniger (1959) Social-cultural background of the aging individual. In J. E. Birren, (ed.), *Handbook of Aging and the Individual.* Chicago: the University of Chicago Press.

Waddington, C. H. (1962) *New Patterns in Genetics and Development.* New York: Columbia University Press.

Wallon, H., E. Evart-Chmielniski, and R. Sauterey (1958) Equilibre statique, équilibre en mouvement: double latéralisation. *Enfance,* 11:1-29.

Watson, J. B. (1919) *Psychology from the Standpoint of a Behaviorist.* Philadelphia: Lippincott, and Co.

Wayner, M. J., and R. Emmers (1958) Spinal synaptic delay in young and aged rats. *Am. J. Physiol.,* 194:403-405.

Webb, W. B., and H. W. Agnew (1962) Sleep deprivation, age, and exhaustion time in the rat. *Science,* 136(3522):1122.

Weiss, L. A. (1934) Differential variations in the amount of activity of newborn infants under continuous light and sound stimulation. *Univ. Iowa Stud. Child Welfare,* 9:1-74.

Weiss, P. A. (1936) Selectivity controlling the central-peripheral relations in the nervous system. *Biol. Rev.,* 11:494-531.

_____ (1937a) Further experimental investigations on the phenomenon of homologous response in transplanted amphibian limbs. I. Functional observations. *J. comp. Neurol.,* 66:181-209.

_____ (1937b) Further experimental investigations on the phenomenon of homologous response in transplanted amphibian limbs. II. Nerve regeneration and the innervation of transplanted limbs. *J. comp. Neurol.,* 66:481-535.

_____ (1937c) Further experimental investigations on the phenomenon of homologous response in transplanted amphibian limbs. III. Homologous response in the absence of sensory innervation. *J. comp. Neurol.,* 66:537-548.

_____ (1941a) Nerve patterns: The mechanics of nerve growth. *Third Growth Symposium,* 5:163-203.

_____ (1941b) Self-differentiation of the basic patterns of coordination. *Comp. Psychol. Monogr.,* 17:1-96.

_____, and M. Edds (1945) Sensory-motor nerve crosses in the rat. *J. Neurophysiol.,* 8:173-194.

Welford, Alan T. (1959) Psychomotor performance. In J. E. Birren, (ed.), *Handbook of Aging and the Individual.* Chicago: the University of Chicago Press.

Wellman, B. L. (1937) Motor achievements of preschool children. *Child. Educ.,* 13:311-316.

Wetzel, N. C. (1941) Physical fitness in terms of physique, development and basal metabolism. *J. Amer. Med. Assoc.,* 116:1187-1195.

_____ (1943) Assessing the physical condition of children: I. Case demonstration of failing growth and the determination of "par" by the grid method. II. Simple malnutrition: A problem of failing growth and development. III. The components of physical status and physical progress and their evaluation. *J. Pediat.*, 22:82-110, 208-225, 329-361.

Whittle, H. D. (1961) Effects of elementary school physical education upon aspects of physical, motor, and personality development. *Res. Quart.*, 32:249-260.

Wild, Monica R. (1938) The behavior pattern of throwing and some observations concerning its course of development in children. *Res. Quart.*, 9(3):20-24.

Williams, J. W. (1931) *Obstetrics.* New York: Appleton-Century-Crofts.

Wilson, D. C., and I. Sutherland (1950) Further observations on the age of the menarche. *Brit. med. J.*, 2:862-866.

————, and ———— (1953) The age of menarche in the tropics. *Brit. med. J.*, 2:607-608.

Wilson, M. U. (1957) Biological changes in American women in the last fifty years. *Res. Quart.*, 28(4):413-421.

Wilson, V. J. (1966) Inhibition in the central nervous system. *Sci. Amer.* 214(5):102-110.

Winchester, A. M. (1961) *Heredity: An Introduction to Genetics.* New York: Barnes & Noble, Inc.

Windle, W. F. (1941) Physiology and anatomy of the respiratory system in the fetus and newborn infant. *J. Pediat.*, 19:437-444.

————, and J. E. Fitzgerald (1937) Development of the spinal reflex mechanism in human embryos. *J. comp. Neurol.*, 67:493-509.

Woolf, Charles M. (1963) Paternal age effect for cleft lip and palate. *Amer. Jour. Human Genet.*, 15(4):389-393.

Woyciechowski, B. (1928) Ruchy zarodka ludzkiego 42 mm. *Polsk. Gazeta Lekarska,* 7:409-411.

Yarmolenko, A. (1933) The motor sphere of school age children. *J. Genet. Psychol.*, 42:298-318.

Yerkes, R. M., and D. Bloomfield (1910) Do kittens instinctively kill mice? *Psychol. Bull.*, 7:253-263.

Younger, L. (1959) A comparison of reaction and movement times of women athletes and non-athletes. *Res. Quart.*, 30(3):349-355.

Zimmerman, Helen M. (1956) Characteristic likenesses and differences between skilled and non-skilled performance of standing broad jump. *Res. Quart.*, 27:352-362.

INDEX